Arthritis

by Ruth Adams
and
Frank Murray

Larchmont Books
New York

First printing: June, 1979

ARTHRITIS

Copyright © Larchmont Books, 1979

ISBN 0-915962-28-4

Printed in the United States of America

LARCHMONT BOOKS
6 East 43rd Street
New York, N.Y. 10017
Tel., 212-949-0800

Contents

CHAPTER 1

Arthritis:
A National Menace

ON NOVEMBER 28, 1976, actress Rosalind Russell died at her home in Beverly Hills, California. She was 63. Although her death was attributed to cancer, the exuberant star of stage and films had been forced to retire from show business some 10 years before because of crippling arthritis.

In her autobiography, *Life Is a Banquet* (Random House, New York, 1977, published posthumously), Miss Russell acknowledged that the last years of her life had been difficult ones. ". . . my arthritis is worse," she said. "I'd be hobbled if I didn't stay on steroids—sometimes the cortisone puffs up my face, giving me chipmunk cheeks—and even with the steroids, my right hip got so bad in August of 1976 I had to have a complete hip replacement." At another point she reported that, once when her husband found her she was not sleeping but was in a coma. "The medicine I'd been taking for my arthritis had concealed the symptoms—steroids do mask symptoms—of pneumonia."

In the preface of the book, her husband, Frederick Brisson, the producer, reported that Miss Russell had had a second mastectomy in 1965, and that in 1969 she was hit by severe rheumatoid arthritis, "for which she started to take

5

medicines which have dangerous side effects." In April of 1975 she contracted pneumonia, the symptoms of which were masked by these medications, he said. And in the fall of 1975 the cancer returned.

Miss Russell, who scored Broadway triumphs in *Auntie Mame* and *Wonderful Town* following a spectacular Hollywood film career, was a vegetarian. She was a heavy smoker during much of her life, she consumed a moderate amount of alcoholic beverages, and she was apparently fond of sweets such as hot chocolate. Her indefatigability was very much in evidence during the grueling months and years of her Broadway successes, but she was often noticeably tired. "That second *Auntie Mame* winter I had the flu three times myself, took antibiotics like popcorn, and kept going," she says in the book. It is not known what effect, if any, these indiscretions had on her health.

She also said that, "When you've got arthritis, your adrenal gland (sic) doesn't work properly. Steroids stimulate the adrenal gland, which is connected with the pituitary gland, which goes to the brain. So you can get euphoric on steroids. And you can turn into a bleeder because of steroids. . . ." (Her editor should have been more accurate about human anatomy, especially that there are two adrenal glands, located above the kidneys, which secrete at least two hormones, adrenalin and cortin).

During her spare time, Miss Russell devoted her considerable energies to the charitable organizations which are trying to find a cure for arthritis. Unfortunately, The Establishment's idea of a cure is to develop new and powerful drugs, each with side effects as long as your arm. Wouldn't it be ironic if the partial answer to Miss Russell's problems—as well as those of millions of cancer and arthritic victims—can be found in their kitchens, dining rooms and living rooms, rather than in the laboratories of the multi-million-dollar drug companies?

ARTHRITIS: A NATIONAL MENACE

As we were completing this book, we attended a press conference by a very courageous doctor of veterinary medicine who believes that he has found a possible clue to cystic fibrosis. The discovery came accidentally while he was autopsying some rhesus monkeys. His theory is that human cystic fibrosis may begin in the fetus, when the human mother is unable to deliver essential nutrients to the developing baby, either because of her metabolism or because she is not getting these nutrients in her own diet. He mentioned the trace minerals selenium and zinc, vitamin E, vitamin B2 and others as being involved in a rather complicated enzymatic process. In New York City, the nation's media capital, only eight or ten reporters turned out for the press conference. Already, the experts on cystic fibrosis are throwing cold water on this theory, without bothering to test it.

Our somewhat cynical opinion is that the government and private foundations are not really interested in finding a cure for arthritis, cystic fibrosis, heart disease, etc. They are not about to kill the goose that lays the golden eggs. If they were to accidentally stumble on a cure, there would go millions of dollars in research grants, big salaries, expensive luncheons and banquets, etc. We already know that heart disease is largely caused by one's own smoking, drinking, eating and exercise habits. We know that cancer is caused by smoking and environmental pollutants to a great extent. And yet millions of dollars continue to be spent on questionable drugs, with little or no thought given to diet, nutrition and environmental factors.

In the July 12, 1977 issue of *The New York Times,* Dr. Christiaan Barnard, one of the world's foremost heart surgeons, was quoted during a Cincinnati, Ohio press conference as saying that he would have to retire within a year or two because of crippling arthritis. "I have great trouble with my hands; I can't continue much longer," the renowned South African physician said.

Arthritis—or rheumatism as it is sometimes called—will affect most of us during our lifetime. We offer in this book a nutritional alternative to the countless arthritic drugs, which are often ineffective and leave disastrous side effects. Our theories can be used by you and your physician by themselves or in conjunction with whatever therapy he or she prescribes.

CHAPTER 2

The Scope of
the Disease

ARTHRITIS SHOWS no mercy, selecting its victims from all walks of life. The disease, in its various forms, is probably the most widespread, crippling, disabling and often painful disease in the United States and probably in the world. "In one way or another, it directly or indirectly affects every American," says *Arthritis: Out of the Maze* (DHEW Publication No. (NIH) 76-1150), published in April, 1976 by the National Commission on Arthritis and Related Musculoskeletal Diseases, Bethesda, Maryland.

The total number of persons with arthritis is unknown, and the statistics we have are limited and out of date. However, according to one nationwide study conducted by the Health Interview Survey in 1969, 10.3 per cent of the population reported having one of the major forms during the preceding year. This suggests that at least 22 million Americans now suffer from arthritis, the just mentioned publication reports.

This figure does not include related musculoskeletal conditions that afflict another estimated six million people, the publication said. "It should be emphasized that these are conservative figures because the household survey on which they are based did not include those in nursing homes, extended care facilities, and similar institutions—many of whom were elderly and likely to be afflicted with arthritis. It also did not include diffuse diseases of connective tissue such as systemic lupus erythematosus."

According to this report, the chances of developing arthritis increase dramatically with age. Approximately five percent of persons between the ages of 17 and 44 have arthritis, compared to 23 per cent for persons between 45 and 64, and 41 percent for people 65 and over.

"Arthritis, however, knows no age limitations," the publication says. "Tens or even hundreds of thousands of parents have watched their young children suffer excruciating pain and limb deformities, sometimes to recover but sometimes doomed to a life of pain, frustration and agony, sometimes faced with blindness, and sometimes fated to early death."

It is probably true to say that most Americans do not realize that the diseases involved in arthritis may affect not merely bones and joints, but also blood vessels, the kidneys, the skin, the eyes and the brain. Arthritis can be a serious result of many infections, including tuberculosis, syphilis, gonorrhea, streptococcal infections, measles and mumps. In some types of arthritis, the complications may result in death.

The prevalence of arthritis and the other musculoskeletal diseases varies by sex as well as age. It is generally more common in women than in men, although in the case of gout the opposite is true. For related musculoskeletal conditions, the prevalence rates for men and women are about the same.

Surprisingly, arthritis is more prevalent in rural areas than in large towns and cities, the HEW publication reports. Most arthritic diseases are more frequent in low-income, low-education groups, while the prevalence of gout is slightly higher in high-income groups. Certain occupational groups—for instance, farmers, workers in heavy industry, and athletes—are known to be more susceptible than are others to degenerative joint disease (osteoarthritis), the publication points out. Although the booklet does not mention it, it is logical to assume that, say, a baseball pitcher, is likely to develop some form of arthritis because of the stress his arm is subjected to during the long pre-season and season. Or take the punishment that a football player is forced to withstand during the season. A farmer or a worker in heavy industry must encounter stress of a different kind: long hours, punishing demands on his body, and perhaps quickie meals that do not offer optimum nutrition.

Which brings us to the low-income groups. For some undefinable reasons, the learned National Commission on Arthritis and Related Musculoskeletal Diseases and its parent bureaucracy—the U.S. Department of Health, Education and Welfare—does not associate arthritis with the below-standard diets that many low-income people subsist on. Even if they are getting food stamps, they may not be nutritionally wise enough to avoid the junk food traps at the supermarket.

The cost of arthritis to Americans may be measured by many yardsticks, the HEW publication goes on. One, of course, is its impact on the national economy. According to estimates of The Arthritis Foundation, the cost for arthritis in 1975 reached a staggering $13 billion.

During 1975, more than $4 billion in wages were lost because of arthritis disability or the inability of arthritis patients to be employed. More than $1.3 billion were involved in losses in homemaker services. Disability insurance payments and aid to those arthritis patients permanently and totally disabled were $1 billion.

The total cost in lost tax revenue to Federal, state and local governments amounted to $955 million. Hospitaliza-

ARTHRITIS

tion for arthritis victims cost another $1.5 billion. Approximately 34.4 million visits to physicians cost arthritis patients $859 million. And prescription drugs cost these patients $690 million. Another $575 million were allocated for nonprescription drugs.

Rehabilitation services, physical therapy, and other care provided by allied health professionals cost $70 million. Unfortunately, few of these services were covered by health insurance or other third-party programs.

Compensation and disability payments by the Veterans Administration for arthritis totaled nearly $427 million. And through the National Institutes of Health, the Federal government spent more than $33 million on arthritis-related research. Other Federal agencies and private foundations spent more than $31 million on arthritis research and treatment projects. Nearly $270 million in earnings were lost because of premature deaths.

The publication says that $484 million were spent on what it calls "quack remedies and devices." The booklet does not say, but some of these remedies may have worked, although, admittedly, arthritis victims, in a vain attempt to relieve their suffering, are easy prey for unscrupulous promoters. But, not surprisingly, we doubt that the affluent Federal and private agencies spent $1.00 on the possible relation between diet and arthritis.

Of course, the magnitude of the problem is more shocking when one recognizes the devastating effects arthritis has on human beings. Here are some of the gruesome statistics:

1.) Arthritis causes more prolonged pain to more Americans than any other disease. More than 5 million people report they are afflicted all the time by their condition.

2.) More than a million people with arthritis and related musculoskeletal conditions are totally disabled and

12

another 2.5 million are partially disabled.

3.) Arthritis resulted in more than 70 million days spent in bed during the past year.

4.) More than nine million people with arthritis went to a doctor for treatment of their condition within the past year. Some 500,000 required hospitalization.

The more personal tragedies can only be spotlighted by case histories. Here are a few, as reported by the HEW booklet.

Case No. 1. "I guess I was 13 when it started. There was this excruciating pain and swelling of the joints in both feet and my left shoulder. It got to the point I couldn't put on my shoes, and my arm froze in an upright position ... I had to drop out of sports, and couldn't get a job like the rest of the kids ... You lose all self-confidence ... You just withdraw from things...."

Case No. 2. "Can you imagine the terrible frustrations of taking our little boy from one doctor to another, trying to find why he had his aches all the time, and his fever, and that little limp ... They finally diagnosed it, and started treatment, but it didn't help ... He died when he was only five years old."

Case No. 3. "It's very hard to try to explain to anyone all of the trials and tribulations an arthritic and her family goes through. There've been many, many days in those 11 years when I had to struggle to get up and do only the very most necessary duties around the house. And, of course, lots of days when I just couldn't do that much."

Case No. 4. "It's not just the pain. All your leisure time activities are pretty much cancelled. You just don't have the energy ... You feel very isolated, and very much alone."

Case No. 5. "It's maddening to find a doctor who would understand my disease, and not just look at my swollen joints and ask, 'Have you tried aspirin?' Or one who'd hand out steroids like popcorn and never mention the side effects."

A more grim case history is given, that of a 27-year-old attorney who, in 1957, three years out of law school, developed the first signs of rheumatoid arthritis. He received treatment but without significant help. At the end of two years, he could hardly walk. Following surgical operations on both knees, anti-arthritis drugs and other treatments, he was eventually able to resume his law practice . . . in 1967. The cost in money alone of this 10-year ordeal is not given.

This brings us to the various forms of arthritis, which are often lumped under the one-word umbrella of "Arthritis." Actually, there are some 80 separate diseases classified as arthritis and related musculoskeletal diseases. New forms are constantly being identified, and the list undergoes frequent reclassification. Some forms of the disease are extremely rare and afflict only a few victims, although some of these lead inexorably to death. Other forms affect millions of people. Most of these forms are difficult to diagnose in their early stages, and a few are difficult to diagnose at any stage.

"The cause or causes of almost all types of arthritis are yet unknown, just as there are, with rare exceptions, no known methods of prevention or cure. In certain forms, palliative treatment is available for most patients, but this palliation may lose its efficacy after a time, or the control methods themselves may cause serious side effects or even death," the HEW publication notes.

CHAPTER 3

The Different Kinds of Arthritis

ACCORDING TO *Arthritis: Out of the Maze,* here are definitions of the more common types of arthritis.

Rheumatoid arthritis. A severely painful and crippling form of the disease, rheumatoid arthritis strikes three times as many women as men. It is relatively uncommon among young adults but becomes increasingly frequent at older ages. However, for those afflicted, nearly half showed signs of the disease before the age of 45. It can be mild or relentlessly progressive and deforming. It is marked by chronic inflammation and overgrowth of the joint linings, erosion of bone, and destruction of the cartilage that normally provides a smooth cushion over the joint surfaces.

The onset may come suddenly, or the disease may develop gradually. Often, it disappears for periods of a few months then flares again. In some fortunate patients, it seems to have vanished for years. It can affect not only a few particular joints, but also organs such as the heart and lungs. The symptoms—fatigue, depression, soreness, stiffness and aching pain—affect the entire body, making it difficult or impossible to hold a job, carry on normal family life, or be a productive member of society.

ARTHRITIS

Some researchers maintain that rheumatoid arthritis, if it is severe enough to require hospitalization, tends to reduce life expectancy, although death is not attributed to it, reports *Arthritis,* Public Health Service Publication No. 1431, April, 1966. Several surveys of hospitalized patients show, for example, that in Boston, 583 rheumatoid arthritis patients, who were hospitalized at Massachusetts General Hospital, were followed for an average of 10 years. There were 257 men and 326 women. During the follow-up period, 137 died. The death rate among males and females who were less than 50 years of age was higher than expected. For males, the difference was striking—about five times greater. The observed rate was 20.6 per 1,000 patient years of observation. The expected rate was 3.9. Among females, the rate was approximately 3½ times that expected (10.7 and 2.9). The investigators reported that the rate differences between the two sexes could be attributed neither to age distribution nor to the spondylitis that was found among the males. For those with rheumatoid arthritis who were 50 years of age or older, mortality rates did not differ too much from that expected in the general population.

Spondylitis—also known as ankylosing spondylitis, Marie's disease, Strümpell-Marie or Marie-Strümpell disease—is caused by an inflammation of one or more of the vertebrae. It is, in essence, arthritis of the spine.

In another study, 275 patients with rheumatoid arthritis, who were admitted to Northern General Hospital, Edinburgh, Scotland, from June, 1948 to July, 1951, were followed for about nine years. These patients were older on the average than those in the Massachusetts study. During the nine-year follow-up period, 75 of the 275 patients died. Mortality rates were reported to be excessive at all ages for these patients. Also, mortality rates were found to be greatest among those that were most severely affected.

THE DIFFERENT KINDS OF ARTHRITIS

Although the Edinburgh patients were an older group, both studies support, in general, the contention that if rheumatoid arthritis is severe enough to require hospitalization, life expectancy is shortened.

Osteoarthritis. Known to physicians as degenerative joint disease, or commonly as "wear-and-tear" arthritis, osteoarthritis is the most widespread form of the arthritic diseases. It is a slowly progressive disorder characterized by a breakdown of cartilage and changes in the bone. Most commonly, it develops in the fingers and in the weight-bearing joints—the knees, the hips, and the spine.

Osteoarthritis can also cause intense pain, deformity and disability. Its frequency increases with age. It can, however, be accelerated by certain occupational stresses that affect particular joints, especially in workers in heavy industry and athletes. Similarly, it can strike victims of automobile and sports accidents.

One study of osteoarthritis based on X-ray examination of the hands and feet disclosed that, among Americans between the ages of 18 and 79, 37 of every 100 had joint changes associated with the disease. In older people, the figures were dramatic—87 per cent of the women and 78 per cent of the men over the age of 65 showed X-ray evidence of the condition. Although as many as 50 per cent of radiologically abnormal joints may cause no symptoms, osteoarthritis is an important source of disability.

According to *Arthritis,* osteoarthritis is reported to be the most common form of the disease that is treated at clinics. Yet, it has been found that as high as 75 per cent of those with osteoarthritis are symptom-free.

Among the studies done in the United States, one provides radiological evidence of osteoarthritis of the hands and wrists among Alaskan Eskimos. The data were compared to similar information that was obtained from examinations of a sample of white persons in the U.S.

ARTHRITIS

Thirteen per cent of the Eskimos, as compared to 24 per cent of the white persons, were reported to have osteoarthritis of the hands. In both groups, the condition was found to be more prevalent above the age of 50. Osteoarthritis was not found among the Eskimos before the age of 30; however, white persons were affected at earlier years.

Evidence from Manchester, England indicates that occupation may influence the development of osteoarthritis. It was five times more common in the knees of underground mine-roadway workers than in those of office workers. Likewise, osteoarthritis of the elbows was more frequent in dockworkers and in miners, especially those who operated pneumatic drills.

Certain joints of the fingers and hands of cotton mill workers were affected more frequently than the same joints in those who had never worked in a cotton mill. Otherwise, the presence of osteoarthritis or disc degeneration differed little between the two groups. Within the mills, differences were noted according to the type of work that was performed. Joints in the fingers of spinners were affected more frequently than those in weavers or card-room workers. An interesting finding of this study was that, although cotton mill workers had more arthritis, they exhibited fewer symptoms than did those who had never worked in a cotton mill, *Arthritis* states.

According to another government publication, *How to Cope with Arthritis* (DHEW Publication No. (NIH) 76-1092, 1977), osteoarthritis may result from overweight, poor posture, injury or strain from one's occupation or recreation, or a combination of these factors.

"The disease is characterized by degeneration of joint cartilage which lines the outside of bones where they move against each other," the booklet reports. "This cartilage becomes soft and wears unevenly. In some areas, it may wear away completely, exposing the underlying bone and damaging it. Disability most often results from disease in the weight-bearing joints. . . . The common symptoms are pain and stiffness. Pain is usually experienced when certain joints are used, especially finger joints and those that bear the body's weight. Enlargement of the fingers at the last joint often occurs. Such enlargements are common and are called Heberden's nodes. Although permanent, enlargements of this type seldom lead to disability."

Arthritis in children. Juvenile rheumatoid arthritis and other forms of rheumatic disease cause significant crippling in children under the age of 18. They can retard growth, cause serious social or emotional problems, and lead to severe kidney disease, blindness or death.

In some young people, these disorders are characterized by fever, rash and mild joint pains; in others by fever and pain in only a few joints, and still others by pain in just one joint. For many, the disease is marked by repeated remissions and flare-ups. Some children seem to "outgrow" the condition, and the symptoms disappear. Others are afflicted throughout life. Approximately 230,000 children suffer from arthritis and other musculoskeletal diseases, not including those who may have entered a remission period.

Systemic Lupus Erythematosus (SLE or Lupus). One of the forms of arthritis that can affect the joints and also the vital organs of the body is Lupus. Others generally placed in the same group of systemic diseases are scleroderma, polymyositis, dermatomyositis and forms of vasculitis. They may be disabling and can be fatal.

Little is known about the cause and nature of these diseases, or even how many individuals are afflicted. Limited studies show that Lupus strikes seven times as many women as men and it afflicts black women three times more frequently than white women. It is a disease of connective tissue which produces changes in the structure and functions of the skin, joints and internal organs.

The illness often follows infection, injury or exposure to sunlight, according to *Medigraph Manual,* by Dr. George E. Paley and Herbert C. Rosenthal. It is hard to distinguish from a condition brought on by the use of certain medicines prescribed to control high blood pressure, they report.

Psoriatic arthritis. This disorder affects about 10 per cent of people with psoriasis, the skin disorder. This arthritis closely resembles the rheumatoid type, and it is treated in a similar manner, with special attention to the skin disorder, reports *How to Cope With Arthritis.*

Reiter's syndrome. This is a combination of urethritis (inflammation of the urethra), arthritis and conjunctivitis (inflammation of the delicate membrane that lines the eyelids). It occurs most commonly in young male adults, and usually lasts only a matter of weeks or months.

Bursitis. This is inflammation of a bursa, a small sac containing fluid, which is usually situated between a tendon and the bone over which the tendon glides. "Tennis elbow" and "housemaid's knee" are examples of bursitis.

Fibrositis is the most common rheumatic condition that does not affect the joints directly. It involves pain, stiffness or soreness of fibrous tissue, especially in the coverings of the muscles. Attacks may follow an injury, repeated muscular strain, prolonged mental tension or depression. Fibrositis within the muscles is sometimes called myositis. Lumbago is fibrositis in the lumbar region. The condition may disappear spontaneously or as a result of treatment. It is not a destructive, progressive disease and is not a crippler, we learn from *How to Cope With Arthritis.*

Ankylosing spondylitis. A disease of the spine that usually occurs in young adulthood, and that is far more frequent in men, ankylosing spondylitis commonly begins in the sacroiliac area and in the small joints of the spine. It is also called rheumatoid spondylitis and Marie-Strümpell disease. In any form, it causes low back pain. The affected joints may ankylose, or calcify, and in severe cases, the spine becomes rigid. Pain may range from moderate to severe, and some victims may be largely or totally disabled.

Ankylosing spondylitis was diagnosed in 0.11 per cent of 200,000 medical and surgical patients that were discharged from Veterans Administration Hospitals. Among patients with ulcerative colitis and regional enteritis, the rate was 20 times more frequent than in general medical and surgical patients who were discharged.

In a 30-year study conducted between 1926 and 1955 of 555 patients in New England with chronic ulcerative colitis, rheumatoid spondylitis was diagnosed in 20 men and eight women. In 18 of the group, spondylitis was confined to the sacroiliac joints, as confirmed by X-ray. In a University of Michigan study of 100 persons with chronic ulcerative colitis, six were diagnosed as spondylitic.

Gout. Perhaps the most painful form of arthritis, gout is the most readily controlled in most patients. It results from a defect in body chemistry that leads to high blood levels of uric acid that, in turn, result in the formation and precipitation of needle-like urate crystals in the joints. Usually gout first involves the big toe, but it can occur in other parts of the body. Unlike other forms of arthritis, gout can generally be controlled. The disorder, which may involve genetic factors, afflicts more than a million victims in the United States. Most of them are men.

"Attacks of gout may follow minor injury, excessive eating or drinking, overexercise or surgery," reports *How to Cope With Arthritis.* "Often, attacks, very sudden in onset, occur for no apparent reason, and may last for days or weeks, during which the patient suffers acute pain and tenderness in his affected joints. Between attacks he may be free of symptoms. Many years after the onset, chronic arthritis may set in. Gouty kidney disease and consequent high blood pressure can develop if the condition is not detected and treated in its early stages."

Pseudogout. This term is used for a disorder marked by acute or chronic inflammation and deposition of calcium pyrophosphate crystals in the joints. It occurs in some patients afflicted with chondrocalcinosis, a condition marked by the deposition of calcium in the cartilage. The similarity of crystal-induced inflammation is a currently recognized basis for conceptually associating gout and pseudogout.

Infectious agents in rheumatic diseases. While an infectious agent has long been thought to initiate rheumatoid arthritis and related diseases, there is as yet no convincing evidence to support this hypothesis. Recent advances in the understanding of host-microbe relationships in certain other chronic diseases, however, now provide leads that could be fruitfully pursued.

For example, it seems likely that several diseases of the central nervous system are caused by as yet unidentified virus-like agents and are characterized by progressive destruction of the host tissues. One of these is caused by the production of an aberrant strain of a common virus such as that of measles. Other viruses seem to be implicated in a variety of so-called auto-immune diseases marked by severe tissue destruction. There is, therefore, growing suspicion that such infectious agents may also be involved in rheumatoid arthritis and related disorders.

Infectious arthritis. Some arthritis may be caused by a wide variety of bacteria, fungi and viruses. Among the causative agents are such bacteria as gonococci, staphylococci, pneumococci, streptococci, pseudomonas and tubercle bacilli. A variety of fungi may also cause inflammation of the joints, but this is relatively infrequent. Bacterial or septic arthritis usually develops from the spread of organisms by means of the blood circulation from a primary infection elsewhere. Bacterial arthritis must be recognized early and treated promptly by appropriate antimicrobial therapy.

Arthritis is one of the major manifestations of rheumatic fever, in which the joints are highly painful and inflamed during an active attack. Since the relationship to streptococcal infection has been established, recurrent attacks of rheumatic fever have usually been prevented effectively with prophylactic antimicrobial therapy, we are told by *Arthritis: Out of the Maze.*

As this planet's oldest known chronic illness, multiple arthritis has been detected in the 100-million-year-old skeleton of a platecarpus—a swimming reptile, according to *Arthritis.* Chronic spinal arthritis has been traced to the ape-man of two million years ago, the Java and Lansing men of 500,000 years ago, and the Neanderthal man of 40,000 years ago. Ankylosing spondylitis has been described in the skeleton of a man who lived 3,000 years before Christ, as well as in human skeletons of succeeding centuries. Egyptian mummies and the remains of prehistoric American Indians show evidence of degenerative joint disease. And history reports the existence of numerous baths throughout the Roman Empire for use by arthritis victims. Today, as you travel through the picturesque Bavarian Alps of Germany and Austria, you find a number of large hospitals devoted to the treatment of arthritis.

During the second century, Galen first defined arthritis as including all rheumatic diseases. As popularly used today, arthritis and rheumatism are virtually synonymous.

Garrod introduced the term "rheumatoid arthritis" in England in 1859. But it was not adopted in the United States until 1941, when it replaced the terms "atrophic arthritis" and "chronic infectious arthritis." Only in the early part of the twentieth century was osteoarthritis or degenerative joint disease differentiated from rheumatoid arthritis.

With the exception of heart disease, arthritis leads all chronic diseases in activity limitation. This is true for both sexes, for white and non-white populations, and in all family income categories. As a cause of days of restricted activity and bed disability, arthritis is topped only by heart disease. As a work-loss cause, it is exceeded only by heart disease and ulcers.

If you have arthritis, first see a doctor. Ask him or her pointed questions about any medication or therapy prescribed. As we have learned, some of the drugs prescribed for arthritis have alarming side effects. Some kinds of arthritis can be aggravated by massage or exercise that may be useful in other forms of the disorder.

"Physical therapy administered in a hospital clinic or at home by a visiting therapist is important to patients unable or unwilling to exercise by themselves," reports *How to Cope With Arthritis.* "The therapist may provide various forms of treatment with heat and massage, or teach patients how to exercise joints by moving them through their full range of motion, how to maintain good posture or use self-help devices. The patient can learn everything he needs to know to care for himself at home, whether independently or with the assistance of family members. . . .

"To aid the arthritic person in performing tasks of everyday living—dressing, eating, cooking, writing, etc.— there are numerous simple and inexpensive devices that can be very helpful and can make the difference between self-sufficiency and dependence. Long-handled combs, shoe-horns, kitchen utensils, heightened chairs and toilet seats are just a few examples of these. Attractive clothes, especially designed for arthritic women, without buttons, snaps or hooks are stylish as well as possible to manipulate with stiff swollen joints.

THE DIFFERENT KINDS OF ARTHRITIS

"To give joints added rest and to help keep them straight, they are sometimes splinted during the night and for periods during the day. A secretary, for example, may use a splint on an afflicted wrist, permitting active use of fingers and hands. Canes, crutches, braces and other such devices share the burden of weight and can be used to aid mobility and to protect against injury and disability," the publication says.

The booklet continues by saying that, in the management of arthritis, the physician must consider the whole person. He must treat not only the pain and stiffness in the patient's joints but the anxieties in his mind, taking fully into account his character, background and personal problems. He may suggest a change of jobs or household routine or some other measure to alleviate a stressful situation.

"No factor is more important in the treatment and rehabilitation of the arthritis patient than maintenance of psychological balance under the stressful conditions imposed by the disease," the publication states. "Complex emotional and vocational problems resulting from chronic disability often require the attention of psychologists, social workers and vocational specialists. In the overall management of arthritis, these specialists must work in close cooperation with each other and with the doctors, surgeons, therapists, relatives of the patient and others involved, if best results are to be achieved."

In this government-sponsored publication, diet and nutritional advice are glossed over in one page and a half. "Contrary to popular belief, there is no such thing as a special arthritis diet. In some cases, certain adjustment in normal diet patterns should be made, depending on the type of arthritis you have. But no diet in itself will cure arthritis," the booklet reports.

What the booklet fails to mention is that, since most

people are notoriously ignorant about good nutrition, some sound nutrition advice should have been given. If you smoke and subsist largely on donuts, chocolate ice cream, potato chips, soft drinks, coffee and other junk foods, you are more likely to develop some forms of arthritis. In many places in this book—even in this opening chapter—we have noted that a sluggish digestive system can cause arthritis.

"It is important for the arthritic person to keep off extra pounds, which can mean an extra burden on weight-bearing joints," the booklet continues. "Additional strain on joints frequently increases pain and may speed progress of disease. Also, when you are in pain, you usually do not exercise as much. So watch those calories to keep from gaining weight, and you will probably feel better.

"Patients with rheumatoid arthritis, on the other hand, often lose their appetite. This can lead to becoming underweight, undernourished and anemic. A nutritionist can offer suggestions to tempt your appetite, and point out rich sources of protein and iron which are particularly necessary for rheumatoid arthritis sufferers."

If we were to grade this paragraph for its nutritional acumen, we would have to give it a D-. To be sure protein and iron are important, but so are vitamins A, B complex, C, D and E, as well as magnesium, zinc, calcium and other nutrients mentioned in this book.

"Patients with gout are not generally given special diets," the booklet says. "Many doctors, however, advise their patients to avoid certain foods (liver, kidney, caviar, sweetbreads, etc.) that are usually high in forerunners of uric acid, the chemicals that accumulate in gouty joints. Excessive use of alcoholic beverages and large amounts of fatty foods are also discouraged. If the patient is overweight, he is usually advised to reduce gradually, under medical supervision. Losing weight too quickly can often lead to attacks of gout.

THE DIFFERENT KINDS OF ARTHRITIS

The arthritis patient should get sufficient rest; particularly during periods when joints are painful and inflamed. Proper exercise is also very important. If arthritic joints are not used for some time, they tend to become stiff and permanently limited in motion. Therapeutic exercises, individually prescribed for the specific condition, are essential not only for the maintenance of joint function, but also for strengthening the muscles that support the joints," the booklet says.

On January 7, 1975, U.S. Senator Alan Cranston (D., Calif.) announced that President Ford had signed a bill authored by the California lawmaker to advance a national effort to conquer arthritis. The bill, the National Arthritis Act, calls for a "planned strategy over the next three years for research into the cause, prevention and cure of arthritis, along with analyses of new treatment techniques."

Senator Cranston said the idea of developing a new national attack on arthritis had its origins in a report by "a prestigious group of rheumatologists, orthopedic surgeons and other leaders in the medical profession." It should not surprise readers of this book that the words "diet" and "nutrition" are not mentioned. Senator Cranston listed six major research goals to help find the causes and cures of arthritis:

1). Determination of whether a viral agent is the cause of arthritis and, if so, its identification.

2). Clarification of the involvement of the immune system in the development of rheumatoid arthritis.

3.) Identification of the mechanisms of inflammation, the early manifestation of most forms of arthritis.

4). Improvement of techniques for replacement of hips and other joints.

5). Statistical surveys of arthritis incidence.

6). Effective treatment of arthritis.

Under the law, Congress was scheduled to appropriate

up to $50 million over the next three years in the anti-arthritis fight. That means that, as we are writing this in 1978, the three years have expired. Have you heard of any dramatic breakthroughs during these three years and $50 million later? We haven't and we read more medical and nutritional journals and talk and correspond with more specialists in diet and nutrition than most doctors.

Senator Cranston, although understandably sincere, was quick to restate the old cliché, "Because there is no successful form of treatment, many arthritis sufferers become victims of false cures and quack remedies." We, too, Senator, abhor false cures and quack remedies, but victims of arthritis often go to any extreme to relieve the pain and suffering. Are these so-called quack cures any more a sham than the miseries caused by prescribed drugs which often leave horrendous side effects?

We suspect that the $50 million might as well have been dumped into a gopher hole. The results, if any, no doubt produced more dangerous drugs that most doctors know very little about, and more worthless surveys which duplicate the countless surveys already in the files.

In the meantime, we invite you to consider a nutritional approach to arthritis. If you have arthritis, or are trying to prevent it, we regret to say that we do not have a cure either. As has been reported, arthritis is a very complicated and illusive disorder. What we do offer are possible alternatives to the plethora of noxious arthritic drugs, which you and your physician can investigate alone or in combination with what therapy he is using. We do not know the answers either, but we implore you and your physician to consider our suggestions objectively. All of this material is the result of some 25 years of painstaking research, involving specialists around the world. Many of these researchers are still alive and can be contacted by your physician for follow-up questions.

THE DIFFERENT KINDS OF ARTHRITIS

The use of vitamins, minerals, herbs, amino acids, corrective diet, etc., is not always successful. But oftentimes it is. A trial-and-error attitude must be assumed by both patient and physician. Best of all, there are no deleterious side effects.

Some of the methods border on hokum... and yet they worked. Was it the vitamin, mineral, herb or whatever ...was it an improved diet in which sugar, white flour and junk foods were entirely eliminated...was it a combination of these elements...was it psychological...was it a miracle? We only know that, for someone afflicted with crippling arthritis, some of the suggestions may work. And since these suggestions are harmless, what have you got to lose?

Our only hope is that many of the researchers, physicians and specialists discussed in this book—and many others who may join them—will continue where these reports leave off in an effort to find out once and for all what dietary and nutritional therapy will prevent and/or cure arthritis. We are confident that the ultimate answer lies with these pioneers, rather than with those bureaucrats who are interested only in enlarging the pharmacopoeia with countless new, unproven and questionable drugs.

As we report in this book, many of these prescribed drugs—along with that old stand-by aspirin—often deplete the body of essential nutrients. And these nutrients could be instrumental in either preventing arthritis or in helping the body to mend once the insidious disorder takes over.

We sincerely believe that many of the answers can be found here. We hope that you are one of those who benefits.

CHAPTER 4

Hunting the Cause of Rheumatoid Arthritis

"IS THERE ANYTHING NEW on arthritis?" is a question asked by millions of people around the world. Yes, there are some hopeful findings. We are reporting a variety of new findings in this book.

A most significant development is the chapter on "Arthritis and Rheumatism" in *The Healing Factor, Vitamin C Against Disease*. This book, by Irwin Stone, was published by Grosset and Dunlap in 1972. Dr. Stone is the scientist whose compilation of facts on vitamin C drew the interest of Dr. Linus Pauling several years ago. Dr. Pauling was so impressed with the wealth of material on the subject that he began his own investigations which led to the publication of *Vitamin C and the Common Cold*.

In his book, Dr. Stone reviews a great deal of past research that has been just tantalizingly short of success in the field of using vitamin C for arthritis and rheumatism. Some of the scientists he reports on had success, others failed. Dr. Stone believes that the problem was usually just not using enough of the vitamin. He quotes one specialist who wrote in 1950, "Our observations suggest that ascorbic acid (vitamin C) when administered in sufficient amounts possesses anti-rheumatic activity.... It is possible that individual doses of ascorbic acid of more than one gram (1,000 milligrams) or total daily doses of more than four grams (4,000 milligrams), if found harmless, may prove to be therapeutically even more effective."

Vitamin C has proved to be harmless even in these massive doses. Dr. Stone comments, "If the government agencies and the publicly supported foundations interested in the arthritic diseases had pursued these scant but provocative leads supplied ... in the 1950's, the past two decades may have seen the elimination of these collagen diseases as a major crippler of the population."

A British team of experts in rheumatology reported in 1968 that they had found the cause of rheumatoid arthritis. There were no ifs, ands or buts. The head of a British Institute of Rheumatology made the announcement, adding, "We can safely say a cure is coming, but we don't know when." The cure seems certain to involve two vitamins: vitamin C and vitamin K3. The British Arthritis and Rheumatism Council thought the statement significant enough to double its financial grant to the Institute for the coming year.

The British medics, experimenting with animals, believe that rheumatoid arthritis, the most common form of this ancient malady, is caused by enzymes escaping from the cells of the joint lining. This eats away the cartilage of the joint like acid, they say. In experiments, using tissues from victims of the disease, they found that vitamin C and vitamin K3 seal up the cell walls, enzymes no longer escape and the disease condition improves.

Since the early days of research on vitamin C and scurvy—the disease of vitamin C deficiency—scientists have known that vitamin C is essential for the health of connective tissue—the cement that binds cells together. It is also believed that one function of vitamin C is related to hydrogen. The vitamin apparently supplies hydrogen to cells. The British rheumatologists think that an excess of tissue hydrogen may be one of the reasons for the leakage of enzymes, which they say causes rheumatoid arthritis.

For many years vitamin C has appeared and reappeared in the medical literature on rheumatism, or rheumatoid arthritis. Over and over, victims of this disease have been shown to have low levels of many vitamins in their blood—especially the water-soluble ones—B and C. Early in the 19th century, Reverend Sydney Smith recommended fresh lemon juice as a cure for rheumatism. This was the most abundant source of vitamin C available at the time, although he could not know this, since vitamins were not discovered until about a century later. Some symptoms of rheumatoid arthritis—the pain, the swelling—are also symptoms of scurvy, the classic disease of vitamin C deficiency.

In 1964, two American physicians tried to inject a solution of vitamin C into rheumatic joints to reduce the thick quality of the joint fluid. Previous studies had shown that the fluid becomes less viscous when blood levels of vitamin C are high. Physicians have long known that anemia frequently accompanies the disease. Anemia indicates, of course, lack of iron in the diet, or inability to absorb dietary iron. Vitamin C helps the body to absorb iron. Then, too, a diet in which iron is lacking is quite likely to be a diet in which vitamin C is also lacking.

In a 1962 issue of the *Rhode Island Medical Journal*, Dr. Michael G. Pierik reported on a 69-year-old woman who had suffered from arthritis symptoms for four years, such severe symptoms that she was confined to a wheelchair and had developed many accompanying symptoms. A test of her blood revealed an almost total lack of vitamin C. A check of her past diet revealed that she had lived for years chiefly on tea, toast, cereal and custards—all foods in which there is no vitamin C whatsoever.

For 18 months she had not partaken at all of such foods as meat, vegetables, fruit. This patient was started on a full diet, plus only 50 milligrams of vitamin C daily. Within 19 days she walked out of the hospital free from all symptoms.

Apart from the possibility of actual lack of vitamin C in diet, there are other reasons why victims of arthritis may be lacking in this vitamin. Smoking has been shown to destroy vitamin C in the blood of heavy, long-time smokers. Aspirin, the drug given most widely for arthritis, causes rapid excretion of vitamin C. So do many other drugs: insulin, anti-histamine drugs, ammonium chloride, thiouracil, thyroid medication, 2:4-dinitrophenol, local anesthetics, atropine, cincophen, barbiturates, amidopyrine, adrenaline, chloroform, chloreton, paraldehyde, stilbestrol, estradiol, sulfa drugs and probably many more of the newer drugs.

Aspirin, given to relieve pain and swelling, is prescribed in relatively enormous doses for arthritics. According to the *Journal of the American Medical Association,* October 12, 1964, "The total dose of aspirin should be large and should be well spread through the day. Minimal maintenance in an adult is about 12 tablets (300 milligram tablets) of aspirin daily, an average dose is 14 to 18 tablets and some young adults readily tolerate 24 or more tablets."

In addition to causing loss of vitamin C, doses of aspirin at this level may also cause digestive upsets, potential ulcers, bleeding from the digestive tract, nausea, loss of appetite, vomiting, ringing in the ears and potential deafness. Doctors speak of one's "tolerance" for aspirin, in full recognition of the fact that it may create more symptoms than it cures. But rheumatoid arthritis pain is very great. So the feeling is that massive doses of this drug are warranted.

If lack of vitamin C in cell walls is indeed the cause of rheumatoid arthritis, it seems possible, does it not, that aspirin and other drugs taken in large doses, may be one of the chief reasons why the patient is deficient in vitamin C? So the continual taking of such drugs would almost guarantee that the arthritis victim would never recover.

Two other significant points. Not so long ago, it was thought that rheumatism is caused by infections in other parts of the body. Teeth and tonsils were extracted. Every infection was carefully guarded against. This therapy is no longer popular. Yet it is well known by nutrition scientists that vitamin C is found in large quantities in the white blood cells, whose job is to fight infections. It is known, too, that the vitamin is destroyed in this battle. So could not lack of vitamin C be a very cogent reason why doctors have linked rheumatism with infections.

Another relevant point is that patients with chronic arthritis have inadequate mechanism for dealing with carbohydrate foods, as diabetics do. As long ago as 1920, a study of 400 cases of arthritis demonstrated that these folks should be on diets high in protein, with carbohydrate cut to the bare minimum, in order to keep their sugar-regulating mechanism in proper balance. Dr. Ralph Pemberton confirmed in 1920 that the worse the condition of the individual's blood-sugar regulating apparatus, the worse his arthritis was bound to be.

People who eat diets high in protein, along with fruits and vegetables as their source of carbohydrate, would naturally have more vitamin C at mealtime than those who shun protein foods, fresh fruits and vegetables and live on sweets. So, while the over-abundance of sweets is disrupting their sugar-regulating machinery, the lack of fruits and other vitamin C-rich foods in such a diet is also predestining them to vitamin C deficiency.

In spite of this wealth of information on the relation of diet to the rheumatic diseases, one continues to read, in medically approved statements, words like these from the *JAMA*, "No particular food item or vitamin has been found to be either beneficial or detrimental in rheumatoid arthritis. A well-balanced diet is recommended." Or this, from Borden's *Review of Nutrition Research*, January-March, 1963: "There is no anti-rheumatic vitamin. Neither is there any substantial evidence that patients with arthritis need any additional quantities of vitamins than those recommended for the ordinary well-balanced diet."

This statement follows the revelation that "patients with... rheumatoid arthritis, like patients with many other chronic diseases, frequently have low blood levels of vitamins." Yet this specialist in rheumatology sees no relation between these facts!

Doctors, it appears, must think in terms of one vitamin, one drug, one diet as the miracle cure for any disease. Yet this is just what they are constantly castigating "food faddists" for! *We* are the people who say that the words "an ordinary well-balanced diet" are meaningless to most people today. The lady who lived on tea, toast, cereal and custards undoubtedly thought she was eating a "well-balanced diet." Why not? No one ever told her otherwise.

And how can doctors give rheumatoid arthritis patients 18 tablets of aspirin a day, knowing full well that aspirin causes rapid, extensive loss of vitamin C, and then announce that no rheumatic patient has any need for extra vitamins? What about the vitamin C that the doctor has just destroyed by his aspirin prescription? How is the patient supposed to replace this, unless he takes massive doses of vitamin C daily?

There is much less information available on vitamin K3. We know that vitamin K is essential for proper coagulation of the blood. There are several forms of vitamin K, one of them found chiefly in leafy, green vegetables, liver and soybeans, the other apparently manufactured by the friendly bacteria in the digestive tract. Many people in these modern times have taken antibiotics for one condition or another, so probably do not have enough of these beneficial bacteria left to give them much additional vitamin K.

The day after the original note about the British research appeared in *The New York Times,* another note appeared. Medical "experts" in England expressed skepticism about the possibility that their colleagues had actually found the cause and possible cure of rheumatoid arthritis. This comes as no surprise. The idea that a simple vitamin deficiency might cause such a prevalent and mysterious disease will cause a lot of skepticism among physicians devoted to the proposition that drugs and drugs alone are the answer to any condition of ill-health.

Several years ago, we wrote to the Arthritis and Rheumatism Foundation and to the National Institute of Arthritis and Metabolic Diseases in Washington. We asked them whether anyone anywhere has ever done any large-scale survey of what rheumatoid arthritis patients actually eat, what general patterns of eating they have followed all their lives. Do they, generally speaking, shun fresh foods and enjoy large amounts of sweets?

We received letters expressing wonder that anyone would ask such a question! Of course, no such surveys have ever been done! Why, the amount of time, money and effort needed to conduct such surveys would be prohibitive! They sent us a lot of pamphlets on how hard they are all working to find a cure, and they thanked us for our interest.

So long as no official information to the contrary is available, it seems reasonable to suspect, doesn't it, that victims of rheumatoid arthritis may simply be people who are not getting enough vitamin C and other essential vitamins in their badly planned diets, or people who may have excessive individual needs for certain vitamins? If the British researchers can prove this by curing arthritis patients with a good diet and massive doses of vitamins, we think a small miracle will be accomplished.

Meanwhile, let's do everything we can to prevent such a catastrophe as arthritis in our own families by always including in every meal plenty of those foods which are rich in vitamin C and vitamin K—fresh fruit, chiefly citrus, deep green leafy vegetables (the greener the better), liver, soybeans, rose hips, and all other elements of a good diet.

CHAPTER 5

Some of the New Arthritic Diseases May Be Viral-Caused

IN THE SUMMER OF 1976, a new type of arthritis was reported in Lyme, Connecticut. It came on suddenly, was extremely painful. It lasted for weeks or months and it sometimes returned. Most of the victims were children, living within the same townships, often on the same street.

"It didn't seem too unusual when we heard of the first case," said the mother of one victim. "That was the girl next door who got it about a year and a half ago. She had to be in a wheelchair on her third attack. Then it hit a little girl around the corner. And after that it was the boy down the street."

Joints swelled making walking impossible. The knee was especially afflicted with swelling of several inches. Sometimes a wrist or elbow was involved. Never hands or feet. One case lasted six months. Treatment has included aspirin, draining the swollen joints and, in one case, an operation to remove the inflamed tissue from the knee. No one has apparently contracted any permanent damage to joints.

Public health authorities were called in. Yale University

experts in rheumatic diseases got interested and soon a complete investigation was being conducted in this part of Connecticut. All the victims lived in heavily wooded areas where houses are far apart. There were no cases in cities or towns. In many victims the arthritic attack was preceded by a rash which started in a small red spot and gradually spread into a large red ring.

The arthritis appeared only during the summer months when insects are about. So Yale specialists in insect-borne diseases were called in. They set up traps to catch insects in this area and studied the possibility that some kind of bug might be responsible. Some of the victims remembered being bitten by "some kind of fly." In a wooded area during a wet summer, insects are everywhere and children playing outside are most likely to be bitten.

According to *The New York Times* for July 18, 1976, the experts found nothing that gave them any clues to the nature of the disease which appeared so suddenly then disappeared, only to reappear in many people.

In a September 25, 1976 press release from the National Institutes of Health, it was reported that a Connecticut grantee had identified 51 cases of "Lyme arthritis." The 39 children and 12 adults lived in the Connecticut towns of Lyme, Old Lyme and East Haddam. Two thirds of the patients experienced recurrent attacks, with some patients suffering from as many as 10 recurrences, and, in some, several joints became affected.

"The unique syndrome is distinguished from juvenile rheumatoid arthritis by its short duration of symptoms, high prevalence of affected males, absence of inflammation of the iris and ciliary body, and its geographical and seasonal clustering. Thus far, all cultures and serological tests have failed to point to a specific agent," the NIH said.

Dr. Stephen E. Malawista and his associates believe that further studies of this phenomenon may provide better knowledge of the poorly understood causes and early stages of many other forms of arthritis. They reported their findings at a meeting of the American Rheumatism Association in Chicago, and an account of this report appears in the July 19, 1976 issue of the *Journal of the American Medical Association.*

Now, according to an article in *Medical World News* for February 21, 1977, Yale investigators believe they have some significant evidence that the disease is indeed caused by an insect or spider bite. The nature of the red spot which appears first seems to indicate a bite of some kind. In the blood of victims who have a rash first, then develop arthritis, a certain unnatural protein appears. This protein decreases or disappears when the joint pain and inflammation disappear, suggesting that it must play a part in the disease.

The skin rash from the small red lump on the skin can last from three days to eight weeks. It is usually accompanied by high fever, fatigue and enlargement of lymph glands near the site of the redness. Stiff neck, headache, backache, nausea and vomiting may torment the sufferer.

As word concerning the disease has gone around in the medical community, reports from other parts of New England have come in. One case was reported from Cleveland. The victim had spent the summer in Old Lyme, Connecticut. Doctors fear that the same symptoms may be appearing in many parts of the country and have just not been recognized as a new disease with, possibly, a very obscure cause. Doctors may be diagnosing it as just another case of arthritis.

The *News* article describes two other kinds of arthritis associated apparently with certain viruses. At a recent meeting of the Arthritis Foundation, a University of North Carolina physician described three patients who developed arthritis three to eight days after the onset of a respiratory infection with fever. Large and small joints of the arms and hands were involved, and two of the three patients had an accompanying rash.

The doctor found signs in the patients' blood indicating that a virus caused the disease. He identified the virus as adenovirus No. 7, a very common type which often causes respiratory diseases and conjunctivitis. He thinks, he says, that arthritis associated with this kind of virus may turn out to be a relatively common disease. He studied several more patients and heard from doctors who reported the same symptoms. The disease clears up in about a month, it seems, so experts in rheumatism may not be seeing these patients.

Still a third arthritic condition was described by two Boston professors of medicine. Symptoms were fever, rash, acute arthritis, starting abruptly with no set pattern as to which symptoms might appear first. And the arthritic pain moved around from one joint to another, although the knees were involved in all cases. Dr. Arthur E. Brawer, one of the Boston physicians who is now in private practice in New Jersey, believes that this disorder involves an inflammation of blood vessels or infection with a virus or both.

It's not much comfort to the rest of us to know that these painful, mysterious disorders may suddenly appear out of nowhere, bringing pain, fever and immobility, especially since there is no medical remedy for viral disease, if that's what causes them. If Lyme arthritis is transmitted by an insect and we don't know which insect or how to avoid it, the only remedy seems to be to shut oneself in the house all during the pleasant summer months. And that, of course, none of us should even contemplate.

Not one of the specialists in arthritis, not one of the physicians who treated these patients mentioned the possibility that large doses of vitamin C might inactivate the virus and counteract the virulence of whatever insect or spider bite might have transmitted the Lyme arthritis.

Some physicians who regularly prescribe large doses of vitamin C for viral complaints also use it to detoxify insect bites. Dr. Fred Klenner of North Carolina successfully treats the bites of black widow spiders with massive doses of vitamin C. And he uses it with equal success to treat viral diseases. In very large doses. Dr. Robert Cathcart of Nevada, an orthopedic surgeon, uses large doses of vitamin C for viral diseases like pneumonia, colds, flu, hepatitis, mononucleosis and finds that his patients heal faster.

CHAPTER 6

Vitamin C Conquers Viral Diseases

"IN CASE OF rheumatoid arthritis, some doctors suspect malfunctions of the immune system perhaps triggered by viruses. Indeed, in recent years, researchers have linked at least four different kinds of arthritis in Africa, Asia and Australia to viruses apparently transmitted by mosquitoes. Other types of arthritis may be bacterial in origin or simply the result of stress at certain joints," reports *Time*, June 13, 1977.

In the previous chapter we discuss 51 cases of "Lyme arthritis," a form of arthritis discovered in the Connecticut River Valley which epidemiologic evidence suggests was caused by an insect vector.

There's a doctor in Nevada who says that vitamin C in large enough doses can lick any virus disease around, and he has the facts and figures to prove it. Dr. Robert F. Cathcart III is an orthopedic surgeon who, by all rights, should be interested only in straightening broken bones rather than curing virus diseases.

But five or six years ago Dr. Cathcart began to hear about Linus Pauling and his theories on vitamin C in the prevention of colds.

Dr. Cathcart had always been especially susceptible to

colds and to hay fever, so being a man of open mind, he tried vitamin C in large doses on himself and found that his susceptibility to colds was much decreased and his hay fever improved. He began to try vitamin C treatment on his patients.

In the five years that followed, he has treated 5,000 patients with massive doses of vitamin C with such success that he received a standing ovation when he reported his results to a group of doctors at a meeting of the California Orthomolecular Medical Society.

Dr. Cathcart found that when he had a cold he could take a much larger dose of vitamin C than he could manage when he was perfectly well. Very large doses, when he was well, gave him some diarrhea, he found. Patients reported that they, too, could take only so much vitamin C without getting diarrhea. It varied with every patient and it varied with their state of health. Those who came to Dr. Cathcart suffering the miseries of some viral infection could take astronomically high doses of vitamin C although they could not handle nearly that much when they were well. People suffering from mild colds, from hay fever and from stress found they could take larger doses than when they were well, but not nearly as large doses as the patients with acute viral diseases.

"There's something very important happening when vitamin C in large enough doses gets inside a patient suffering from a viral disease," says Dr. Cathcart. "Nobody understands just what it is or how it works, but it does work."

He has successfully treated cases of flu, infectious mononucleosis, infectious hepatitis, all the infectious children's diseases like measles, chicken pox, mumps as well as shingles and cold sores. The amount needed varies with the disorder and the individual. He has also used it against scarlet fever and bladder infections, penicillin rash, bee stings, poison oak, hangovers, tooth extractions, injuries, urethritis.

The inflammatory disorders are also likely to yield to large enough doses of vitamin C—things like bursitis, tendonitis and even arthritis—usually in cases of very elderly debilitated people. Why? Dr. Cathcart does not know, but this does not prevent him from using the vitamin, especially when it's a disorder for which he might have used cortisone or some relative of cortisone. Doctors are reluctant to use these drugs, he points out, because of the danger of side effects. The vitamin C appears to do the job just as well in many cases, with no side effects.

Dr. Cathcart labels colds as 50-gram colds, 60-gram colds or 100-gram colds. You should take 50 grams (50,000 milligrams) of vitamin C to treat a 50-gram cold, 60 grams for a 60-gram cold and so on. Any smaller amount of the vitamin won't work, he reports. Of course, if you have only a slight cold, you don't need nearly so much. But, he says, some doctor may have been secretly reading Dr. Pauling's books on vitamin C and may decide to try the vitamin for a patient who comes in with a cold. He may recommend 10 grams a day of vitamin C spaced out over the day, every four hours or so. And, if it's a 30-gram cold, it won't be cured. It just wasn't enough vitamin C for that particular cold. So the doctor will decide that vitamin C really doesn't cure colds. And that's not the case. Enough vitamin C would probably have done the trick, but he didn't know how much to give.

You can see from this that it's pretty much up to each of us to find out for ourselves how much vitamin C we need to avoid a lot of unpleasant minor ailments that may bother us from time to time. When or if a cold appears likely, it's up to us to decide on the basis of trial and error just how powerful a cold is threatening and how much vitamin C we may need to fight it off.

ARTHRITIS

We know that vitamin C performs many, many functions inside our bodies, that it takes part in many enzyme systems which control the way we use this or that nutrient, the way our blood cells build up resistance to infections, the way collagen is kept healthy or destroyed. Collagen is the protein substance of which most of our bodies are made—the protein glue that holds us together. The adrenal glands which help to protect us from stress depend on vitamin C for their function. People who are deficient in vitamin C can find that wounds or sores do not heal rapidly. This suggests that taking enough vitamin C will help them to heal much more rapidly.

In addition to the viral diseases, stress makes big demands on our stock of vitamin C. What do we mean by "stress?" Any disease, however slight, is stressful. The more serious the disease, the more stress it brings. Fatigue is stressful. Worry is stressful. The death of a family member or friend, loss of a job, a long and tiring trip, frustration, exposure to noise and pollutants—the list is very long. Exposure to any of these increases your need for vitamin C. It seems possible that the reason we so often get sick after some stressful circumstance may be lack of vitamin C. Perhaps we could prevent it by taking much more vitamin C during the stressful time.

We know that all the animals which make their own vitamin C in their livers (and this includes almost all of them except human beings) make many times more vitamin C when they are under stress. A laboratory rat living the calm, well-nourished life such animals live, makes 4.9 grams of vitamin C in his liver every day to keep healthy. If he is exposed to stresses like noise, cold or great exertion, the amount of vitamin C he manufactures increases to 15.2 grams a day. This suggests that human beings could be more resistant to stress if they would greatly increase their vitamin C intake during such times.

VITAMIN C CONQUERS VIRAL DISEASES

Dr. Cathcart told his physician audience an interesting story about the stress that may be involved in "getting a shot" against some infectious disease. During the swine flu vaccination drive, Dr. Cathcart and his daughter were immunized. They tested their vitamin C status with a dependable tongue test before they got the shots. It indicated that their vitamin C store was in good shape. The day after the shot they tested again and the test showed "negative—vitamin C way down." It remained that way until the redness and soreness disappeared from their arms, then returned to normal. Dr. Cathcart has no explanation for this, he says, but he believes it shows that immunization is a form of stress which makes heavy demands on the body's store of vitamin C.

In very serious viral illness where the patient cannot take enough vitamin C by mouth, Dr. Cathcart gives it intravenously. After an operation, for example, the patient may succumb to pneumonia, perhaps because the stress of the operation used up what little vitamin C might have been available in his body. Giving huge doses of vitamin C intravenously may save the patient's life. Dr. Frederick Klenner of North Carolina, who has been using vitamin C for many years in his practice, gives as much as 10 to 12 grams of vitamin C intravenously every eight hours under such circumstances. Dr. Cathcart has given as much as 215 grams (215,000 milligrams) of the vitamin both by mouth and intravenous drip to one patient, reducing the dosage gradually as the patient threw off the infection and got well.

Dr. Cathcart says that in five years of practice, not a single patient suffering from a viral infection has had to be hospitalized. Vitamin C is the treatment of choice in every instance. Shingles, for example, is the agonizingly painful viral infection of a nerve system. He says it can easily be cured with very large doses of vitamin C. And if these large doses are continued for two weeks the infection will not return. In many cases where nothing but pain-killers are given, it does return and may last for months or years.

How do you know how much vitamin C to take just to stay healthy or to prevent or treat some viral disorder? Adjust your dosage to what Dr. Cathcart calls "bowel tolerance"—that is, increase it until you get diarrhea. If you feel a cold coming on, increase it still further. You may find that you can take much, much more at such a time before having trouble with diarrhea. Stick with this new dose until the cold disappears, then go back to the maintenance doses. And, always, regulate it by your "bowel tolerance."

The dose of vitamin C necessary for an acute viral illness is so high that you can't imagine it, says Dr. Cathcart. Isn't it possible you may have serious after effects? Recent scare stories in the newspapers have suggested—and they crop up in newspaper medical columns every month or so—that large doses of vitamin C may create a deficiency of vitamin B12. Other researchers have said that such doses might create kidney or bladder stones. In all his 5,000 patients, Dr. Cathcart has never seen either of these conditions and, presumably, he has watched closely for any serious side effects. Dr. Klenner has never seen these predicted catastrophes, either.

Dr. Cathcart says he has found that the average person can take as much as 10 to 15 grams (10,000 to 15,000 milligrams) of vitamin C when they are well, with no threat of diarrhea. If they have a slight cold they can take as much as 30 to 50 grams (30,000 to 50,000 milligrams) of vitamin C with no diarrhea. Patients with infectious mononucleosis can easily take as much as 200 grams (200,000 milligrams) daily with no problems.

He believes, he says, that these wide differences in "tolerance" indicate degrees of absorption in the bowel. Well people will absorb as much as they need for good health. If they take too much, some of the vitamin C is not absorbed and creates diarrhea. In the case of illness, the patient needs so much more of the vitamin that every bit of it is absorbed. So the amount of vitamin C you need varies from day to day. If you are beginning to get a cold you will be able to take far more vitamin C than you usually do. Then, too, if you are under stress you will be able to take more than when you are not under stress. No one but you can determine how much you should be taking every day. It's a challenge.

Dr. Cathcart regularly cures bladder infections with massive doses of vitamin C. He has used it successfully to treat scarlet fever, hay fever, insect stings, poison oak. He has treated penicillin reaction with vitamin C. Some forms of arthritis are alleviated with large doses of vitamin C, especially in elderly debilitated patients. He has also used it in bursitis and tendonitis, but you really have to "pour it on" in some cases, he says. One would think that anyone suffering from these excruciatingly painful disorders would not mind "pouring on" the vitamin C if there was a chance of relief.

Yes, vitamin C might help a hangover, Dr. Cathcart thinks, the pain of a tooth extraction or injury or urethritis. Any condition characterized by inflammation may yield to the vitamin. But remember that detoxifying the disease uses up the vitamin rapidly. This is why such large doses must be used.

He believes, he says, that it is most important, right now, for medical research to study in depth the differences between sick people and well people in relation to nutrients and drugs. His own experience with his 5,000 patients has shown him that there is a vast difference in the way sick people and well people react to everything. Doctors must begin to realize that the sicker the patient is, the more vitamin C they must and can use. Giving too little will simply not get results.

CHAPTER 7

Vitamin C and Ankylosing Spondylitis

ACCORDING TO *The Merck Manual,* 12th edition, ankylosing spondylitis (Marie-Strümpell Disease) is "a chronic, progressive disease of the small joints of the spine separable as an entity from rheumatoid arthritis on genetic, epidemiological, pathological, clinical, serologic and therapeutic grounds . . . neither aspirin nor phenylbutazone (butazolidin) can cure or arrest the progressive ankylosis (stiffness of the spine)."

Statistics reveal that one out of every 330 adult men suffer from ankylosing spondylitis. Army doctors have found that it is a frequent cause of backache in soldiers.

In 1964, Norman Cousins, long-time editor of the prestigious *Saturday Review*, flew home from a lengthy, tiring and frustrating trip abroad. His slight fever and general achiness rapidly developed into a stiff neck and back and great difficulty in moving arms, hands, fingers and legs. His doctor hospitalized him when his sedimentation rate reached 80 mm per hour. The sedimentation rate is the rate at which red blood cells settle out of anticoagulated blood. It may indicate an inflammatory condition, an infection or a cancer.

The doctors decided Mr. Cousins had a very serious

collagen disease. This category includes all the arthritic diseases. As the crippling disease progressed, leaving him unable to turn over in bed, the doctors told him he was suffering from ankylosing spondylitis. Spondylitis is inflammation of the vertebrae. Ankylosing means stiffening or locking in place. The patient was faced with eventually being totally unable to move.

Mr. Cousins' doctors told him he had one chance in 500 of recovering; one specialist said he had never personally seen a recovery from as serious a case as this. Mr. Cousins was being given a number of pain killers for the agonizing pain he was suffering. Associates at the *Saturday Review* researched these drugs and reported to him the highly toxic side effects he might expect. Butazolidin and aspirin were the two he was most worried about, for the doctors prescribed massive doses of both these drugs. A test showed that he was allergic to all of them. He was covered with hives and "felt as though my skin was being chewed up by millions of red ants."

Mr. Cousins decided he would stop taking the drugs and somehow get well on his own. His wide reading had acquainted him with many theories on the power of the mind over illness. He knew how terribly destructive to health negative emotions, hopelessness and anxiety can be. He decided he would turn his thoughts to getting well and abandon all negative thinking. He started a program of reading books on humor and laughter and watched comic films sent in by a friend.

Then he remembered his reading about vitamin C. He asked himself, "Couldn't it combat inflammation? Did vitamin C act directly or did it serve as a starter for the body's endocrine (gland) system—in particular, the adrenal glands? Was it possible, I asked myself, that ascorbic acid had a vital role to play in 'feeding' the adrenal glands?"

He had also read that arthritics seem to be deficient in vitamin C. He thought perhaps this might be because the body uses up its supply of vitamin C in fighting the breakdown of collagen which is the connective tissue damaged in these diseases. Fortunately, his doctor was a long-time friend who had a completely open mind about his treatment and was willing to try anything Cousins suggested.

He told his doctor he wanted to take massive doses of vitamin C. His doctor said he thought there might be danger of kidney damage. Cousins was willing to take the risk. The doctor told him that the largest dose of vitamin C ever given in that hospital was three grams (3,000 milligrams) injected into muscle.

Cousins speculated that "introducing the ascorbic acid directly into the bloodstream might make more efficient use of the vitamin, but I wondered about the body's ability to utilize a sudden massive infusion. I knew that one of the great advantages of vitamin C is that the body takes only the amount necessary for its purposes and excretes the rest.... I wondered whether a better procedure than injection would be to administer the ascorbic acid through slow intravenous drip over a period of three or four hours. In this way we could go far beyond the three grams. My hope was to start at 10 grams and then increase the dose daily until we reached 25 grams (25,000 milligrams)."

His doctor was astonished at the suggestion. Again he said he was afraid of kidney damage as well as damage to veins subjected for so long to an intravenous drip. "He said he knew of no data to support the assumption that the body could handle 25 grams over a four-hour period, other than by excreting it rapidly through the urine," says Cousins.

They tested the patient's blood and started the intravenous drip, administering 10 grams the first day. Within four hours the blood test showed a 9-point improvement.

"Seldom had I known such elation," says Cousins. "The ascorbic acid was working. So was laughter. The combination was cutting heavily into whatever poison was attacking the connective tissue. The fever was receding and the pulse was no longer racing."

They increased the amount of vitamin C a little every day until, by the end of the week, Cousins was getting 25 grams in an intravenous drip. By this time he was off all drugs and sleeping pills and was sleeping naturally. By the end of the eighth day he was able to move his thumbs without pain. The blood tests continued to improve. Two weeks later he was able to go south to bathe in the warm ocean. He could stand by himself, walk, even jog a bit. For many months he had pain and stiffness when he lifted his arms, his fingers were less skillful than he wished when he played the organ, he sometimes had difficulty turning his head. But this presumably incurable disease had been conquered without drugs.

Seven years later, in 1971, he found in *The Lancet,* a British medical journal, a study of how aspirin destroys vitamin C in the human body. This, apparently, is one reason why arthritics are generally deficient in the vitamin, since aspirin is the commonest drug used for arthritic pain. "It was no surprise, then," says Cousins, "that I had been able to absorb such massive amounts of ascorbic acid without kidney or other complications."

Norman Cousins' account of his victory over this crippling disease appeared in the conservative *New England Journal of Medicine* for December 23, 1976. In the latter part of his article he speculates on the possibility that vitamin C may have acted as a placebo in his case. A placebo is a pill or treatment which contains nothing of any medical value. But often the patient feels better, believing that the pill is powerful. He believed in vitamin C so thoroughly, he says, that perhaps it was his belief rather than any biological action of the vitamin which brought his blood corpuscles back to normal and took the stiffness from his spine. He discusses the place of placebos in medical treatment and suggests that much more research should be done along these lines.

He describes his visit to the clinic of Dr. Anna Aslan in Rumania, who told him she believes that there is a direct connection between a strong will to live and chemical balances in the brain. She thinks that the will to live stimulates the entire glandular system, thus possibly bringing about "cures" that are otherwise inexplicable. Of course, Dr. Aslan also uses a drug of the novocaine family which breaks down into a B vitamin inside the body. And she gives immense amounts of tender, loving care, security, hope, encouragement and praise to patients in her geriatric (old folks) clinic.

Dr. F. J. Ingelfinger, the distinguished editor of the *New England Journal of Medicine,* wrote an editorial in the same issue as the Cousins article, trying to analyze the incident. He reminded his physician readers that miraculous, unexplained cures take place sometimes in medicine and that complaints about overwhelming the patient with drugs "are as ancient as the drugs themselves."

"Of greatest interest—at least to me," said Dr. Ingelfinger, "is the nature of Mr. Cousins' processes of reasoning as he cures himself by willpower, laughter, vitamin C and self placebotion...here is an astute, perceptive, articulate and distinguished layman who takes his treatment away from the medical establishment and wins out." How does it happen, then, that his doctors were not as familiar as Mr. Cousins was with the possibility of cure from willpower, laughter and the action of vitamin C, whether real or imagined?

"Well," says Dr. Ingelfinger, "when a patient's condition

involves 'a serious collagen illness,' 'adrenal exhaustion,' polypharmacy (lots of drugs), the advantages of a high-fiber diet, and 'allergy tests' for drugs, medical fallibility, perplexity and controversy could hardly be greater; and the latest medical-journal articles on such clinical topics range from pure bunkum to results of experiments that are scientifically unexceptionable but still do no more than nibble away at the margins of vast expanses of ignorance... at present, it is not possible for the medical establishment, any more than for Mr. Cousins, to speak with confidence about collagen disorders, their protean (variable) manifestations and their often unpredictable course."

We are sorry to say we think this is a cop-out, Dr. Ingelfinger. The incident Mr. Cousins describes happened in 1964. In the ensuing 13 years, so far as we can determine, not a single physician made any attempt to use an intravenous drip of vitamin C for arthritic diseases—whether for its real or imagined value. Mr. Cousins reports no side effects. Such a treatment could have done no harm to the thousands, perhaps hundreds of thousands, of agonized patients who have suffered from this condition in those 13 years. Why has not the medical profession, or the National Institute of Health, or the Arthritis Foundation or *somebody* in charge of something experimented further with this harmless therapy, just to see whether they might be able to ease a little pain and stiffness, even if they cannot work the complete miracle Mr. Cousins reports?

Cousins himself says he did not make the story public earlier because he did not want to raise false hopes in other sufferers from these diseases. Every treatment given to a victim of a chronic arthritic disease raises false hopes, Mr. Cousins. Aspirin may control the pain for a while. Then the patient can't tolerate any more aspirin. Butazolidin controls the pain but the side effects may be far more devastating than the disease. So the drug must be discontinued. Cortisone, used to ease pain in many other arthritic diseases, is fraught with perils, including the eventual total destruction of the body's bones. Why would it be unethical to "raise false hopes" by giving the patient a completely harmless treatment?

As Mr. Cousins points out plaintively, someone in a hospital is always sticking needles into patients for one purpose or another. Intravenous administration of drugs is quite common. Why, then, not try intravenous administration of a harmless vitamin? We cannot help but feel that the answer has nothing to do with the confusion of the medical profession over methods of treatment of collagen diseases. It has to do rather with the fact that most doctors learn what they know of medical therapy from drug salesmen. No drug salesmen are selling vitamin C. It can't be patented. It costs next to nothing. No money-hungry drug company wants to bother with it.

Vitamin C is intimately concerned with the manufacture and the health of collagen—the connective tissue which ties all parts of the body together. If you are suffering from one or another of the chronic, extremely painful and disabling collagen (arthritic) diseases, why not get a copy of Mr. Cousins' article and show it to your doctor or ask him to read the article in his medical library. Do you see any reason for not taking advantage of this therapy, especially if you believe in the helpfulness and beneficence of vitamin C, as Mr. Cousins did?

Several letters from physicians were later published in the *New England Journal of Medicine.* They spoke only of the value of "placebo," laughter and "the will to live." They said that any effect of the vitamin C was that Cousins had faith in it. "We ought to do more studies of 'the placebo effect,'" they said. Not a single physician indicated that he believed the massive vitamin C injections had any effect.

VITAMIN C AND ANKYLOSING SPONDYLITIS

But the letters that came to Norman Cousins were different, he says in an article in *Saturday Review* for February 18, 1978. He says that most of the letters indicated "evidence of an open attitude by doctors to new or unconventional approaches to the treatment of serious disease. There was abundant support for the measures that had figured in my own recovery—a well-developed will to live, laughter and large intravenous doses of sodium ascorbate (one form of vitamin C). Far from resenting the intrusion of a layman into problems of diagnosis and therapy, the doctors who wrote in response to the article warmly endorsed the idea of a patient's partnership with his physician in the search for a cure."

He tells two stories of laymen who got in touch with him which would be unbelievable except that most of us have had similar experiences with doctors. One, a lawyer with a 4-year-old daughter dying of viral encephalitis, asked his doctor about giving the child vitamin C in massive doses. The doctor told him this was nonsense and he didn't welcome instructions from a layman.

So the lawyer bought a pound of powdered sodium ascorbate (which has a slightly salty taste, but not a sour taste). He asked the doctor if he might give his little girl some ice cream. The doctor said certainly. So the next day the little girl got a dish of ice cream laced with 10 grams (10,000 milligrams) of vitamin C. The next day the dose of vitamin C was larger, and the next larger still. The child continued to eat the ice cream. Two weeks later she was well enough to be removed from the oxygen tent. She was completely recovered when the lawyer last reported to Cousins. He had been giving her 25 grams (25,000 milligrams) of sodium ascorbate in her ice cream every day without the doctor's knowledge.

A Boston woman phoned Cousins about her husband, a terminal cancer patient who had been through the standard treatment—radiation, surgery and chemotherapy. She was very concerned about his condition. Cousins said he could not offer any advice since he was a layman, but he told her of the experiments of Dr. Ewan Cameron of Scotland, who has been giving terminal cancer patients large doses of vitamin C as their only treatment and comparing their condition to that of other similar patients getting orthodox treatment. There is no question that the patients treated with vitamin C have less pain, can conduct their lives almost normally, and most of them, live much longer pain-free lives than the patients not so treated.

The woman asked her doctor about giving vitamin C to her husband. He answered with a "quack, quack" and told her the entire business was tommyrot. She and her husband severed their relationship with their doctor, although he was a longtime friend. The cancer patient moved home from the hospital and has gained some ground. "His appetite has improved; and so has his will to live," says Cousins. "He has already had a few more months of life than seemed possible only a short time ago."

Many of the 3,000 physicians who wrote to Cousins spoke of the value of faith in one's doctor and one's treatment, and speculated that it was Cousins' will to live, rather than the vitamin C which caused his almost miraculous recovery. But some of the 3,000 physicians said "don't you believe it was just faith and the will to live which worked this miracle." Two Illinois researchers told him their extensive research had showed the effects of vitamin C on red blood cells which apparently restores the body's "balance" or "homeostasis."

Other testimony came from Lederle Laboratories where scientists are working on the effects of vitamin C on a body enzyme which must have lots of vitamin C to function properly. This enzyme is responsible for the health of collagen, which is the substance that breaks down and becomes diseased in the "collagen diseases"—including all those related to arthritis.

Says Cousins, "One can understand the apprehensions of the medical profession about the absurd notion that vitamins are the answer to any illness. Yet it is also true that some doctors have fostered the equally erroneous idea that the average supermarket shopping basket is insurance against any nutritional deficiency. Considering the preservatives, coloring agents, additives, and sugar overload in many processed foods, the pronouncement of the White House Conference on Food, Nutrition and Health in 1969 seems highly pertinent; namely, that one of the great failures in the education of medical students is the absence of adequate instruction in nutrition. . . . It is worth calling attention to the current practice of many British hospitals of administering intravenous doses of ascorbic acid instead of antibiotics as a routine postoperative procedure in guarding against infection."

Cousins does not underestimate the value of "will to live." He tells us when he was a child he spent many months in a tuberculosis sanitarium where he and a number of other young folks were determined to overcome their disease. They were cheerful and got involved in many interesting activities. Many of their group were dismissed as cured, whereas those who had given up did not respond nearly as well to treatment.

Cousins also tells us of an insurance company's doctor who told him in 1954 that he had suffered a serious heart attack and must give up all his activities and go to bed. Without even consulting his wife or his doctor, Cousins decided he would not accept this recommendation and that he would, instead, get all the exercise he could. His doctor agreed with him when Cousins explained his viewpoint. Years later, Dr. Paul Dudley White told him he had done the only thing that could have saved his life. He believed that sustained and vigorous exercise is necessary for the health of the human heart, "even when there is evidence of the kind of cardiac inefficiency that had been diagnosed in my case," says Cousins.

Cousins also gives a lot of credit to his wife who, he says, has a positive outlook on life and "believes deeply in the advantages of good nutrition."

Ten years after his collagen disease was pronounced incurable by specialists in a leading New York hospital, Cousins met on the street one of the doctors involved in the prognosis. He gave him such a vigorous handshake that the physician winced and asked him to let go. "He said he could tell from my handshake that he didn't have to ask about my health, but he was eager to hear about my recovery."

We suggest a 10-gun salute for Norman Cousins, who has the courage to take on the entire medical establishment and coax from about 3,000 of its members the acknowledgement that laymen should play a large part in deciding on their own treatment, that all of the modern gadgetry of the hospital is useless without faith in the doctor and the treatment he is giving.

Says Cousins, "Hundreds of letters from doctors . . . reflected the view that no medication they could give their patients is as potent as the state of mind that a patient brings to his or her own illness. In this sense, they said, the most valuable service a physician can provide to a patient is helping him mobilize all the resources of mind and body in order to maximize his own recuperative and healing potentialities."

Along with, of course, the judicious use of good nutrition and the preventive and healing powers of those mysterious food elements our doctors know almost nothing about—vitamins and minerals.

CHAPTER 8

Is Rheumatoid Arthritis Related to Allergies?

"THE RECENT PUBLIC DISCLOSURE in the *National Inquirer* (June 7, page 20), that rheumatoid arthritis is caused primarily by food allergy is impressive, based on 20,000 cases treated with 50 to 92 percent success. This has immediately created an immense backlog of food allergy cases whose prompt treatment is vastly beyond current medical capability," says William E. Catterall, Nutritionist, of Tucson, Arizona, in a letter to the editor of *Chemical and Engineering News,* August 1, 1977.

"It is hoped that the medical profession will now rise to the occasion, especially since arthritics have already been abused enough," he says.

Dr. Catterall goes on to tell us that allergists have been reporting food allergy as a cause of this disease for 28 years. He tells us of four cures reported in *Annals of Allergy* in 1949, in spite of supposedly irreversible joint damage. One of these patients was allergic to lettuce, potato and stringbeans, while another had only one allergy—beef.

In 1972, A. Rowe reported on 28 cases of food allergies causing arthritis. These appeared in his book, *Food*

Allergy—Its Manifestations and Control and the Elimination Diets. In 1972 also, M. Millman published "An Allergic Concept of the Etiology (Cause) of Rheumatoid Arthritis," which appeared in *Annals of Allergy,* Volume 30, 135 (1972).

Dr. T. G. Randolph and L. G. Dickey have also presented 200 cases "in a monumental symposium on environmental allergy."

"All these people are allergists," says Dr. Catterall, "who have published their work in sources read primarily by other allergists. Thus there has been a large communication gap, but there has also been a tremendous gap created by provincialism and prejudice. Arthritics deserve better."

One would think that any physician, faced with this baffling and tenacious disease, would be overjoyed to hear that something as "curable" as allergy might be the cause. Therapy in cases of food allergy consists almost entirely of discovering what the offending foods are and then eliminating them from meals and snacks. Granted, this is a long and tiresome business. But isn't it infinitely preferable to enduring the agony of arthritic pain throughout one's life, or the powerful pain drugs whose side effects may be even worse and more destructive?

Isn't it possible, too, that any diet which has been found to alleviate arthritis may be successful because it eliminates those foods to which the arthritis victim is allergic?

In *The Arthritis Handbook*, Darrell C. Crain, M.D. says, "One of the oldest and still widely held views is that this form of arthritis is the result of an infection; but to date no infectious agent has been isolated or proved. Investigators continue to try to discover whether it is a bacterium, a virus, or some organism that may have properties of each of these. It seems possible that the organism would not have to invade the joint itself to produce arthritis. Rather, the joint changes may be due to toxic *or allergic* influences from infection elsewhere in the body."

Later in the same book he tells us that joints will occasionally be involved in a generalized allergic reaction. This happens most often after an injection of something to which the person is allergic—penicillin or tetanus antitoxin, for example. One joint or several may swell rather abruptly and stay that way for several days although there is no pain, "only a feeling of tightness." The patient or the doctor can usually relate the swelling to other allergic symptoms such as giant hives. The swelling responds to antihistamines.

"Some arthritics . . . note that their symptoms are adversely influenced by particular foods," says Dr. Crain. "I have several patients who say that whenever they eat concentrated sweets in the form of chocolate candy they find on the next day that their arthritis is worse. Others report difficulty after taking one or another of the citrus fruits or tomato juice. . . . It is doubtless wise, when an (arthritis) patient has had a bad day, for him to think what food he has eaten during the last 24 hours. If he has had any unusual food, he should give himself a trial period, both on and off this particular food to see if his system seems allergic to it. If so, then he should of course avoid it."

Dr. Sam Roberts, speaking of allergy in general, in his book, *Exhaustion, Causes and Treatment,* tells us that many allergic patients fail to eat a balanced diet and seem to neglect particularly the foods containing vitamin A, the bioflavonoids and vitamin C. "These patients will also deny any aversion to foods high in these vitamins, but their dietary records strongly reveal an inherent perhaps unconscious distaste for most of them. Another significant observation revealed by the dietary histories is the conspicuous tendency of allergic individuals to consume large quantities of refined sugar in foods and beverages, which paradoxically produces a low blood sugar.

"Many allergic children," he goes on, "and some adults consume as much as 30 teaspoonsful of refined sugar each day, some even more. These facts would rarely if ever be discovered without the carefully planned dietary history."

Dr. Roberts puts his allergic patients on diets to correct low blood sugar. The diets are high in protein, and completely eliminate refined carbohydrates—that is, sugar and white flour and everything made from them. In very bad cases, he also gives an extract called *ACE*—adrenal cortical extract—which he gives in smaller and smaller doses until it can be eliminated *after* the exhausted adrenal glands have been restored to good health. He also gives calcium tablets to allergic sufferers.

Strangely enough, Dr. Roberts does not forbid the foods to which the patient has been found to be allergic. Rather than that, he introduces them again in extremely small amounts, increasing this ever so gradually until the patient no longer has any difficulty with the food. For example, if someone is allergic to tomato juice, Dr. Roberts insists that he start with one tablespoonful of tomato juice, then increase the amount gradually every day until six or eight ounces are well tolerated. The same is true of other foods. He says that he has never noted any difficulties in those patients who have had injections of ACE.

The patients whom Dr. Roberts was treating for allergic manifestations (in this case asthma) always had their worst attacks during the night. He reasoned that this must be due to low blood sugar. That is, the attack came on at the moment when blood sugar levels had dropped to their lowest point. He had these patients waken at this time and eat some protein food.

Anyone with arthritis will tell you that pain and stiffness are much worse in the early morning hours. Doesn't it seem possible that low blood sugar may be at least one important reason for arthritis, especially considering the abundant evidence that most arthritics have a life history of being enthusiastic consumers of sweets, especially white sugar products? We have encountered this comment in almost every piece of literature we have read about this disease.

Much evidence also links allergies of all kinds to the functioning of the adrenal glands—those helpful organs that protect us from stress of all kinds. If allergies are one cause of arthritis and if both allergies and arthritis are related to inadequate functioning of the adrenal glands, mightn't it be a good idea to load up on those nutrients which keep the adrenals healthy?

Carlton Fredericks in his book, *Food Facts and Fallacies,* lists the following as food elements essential for the adrenals: the minerals copper, cobalt, manganese, along with vitamin A, the vitamin B complex, vitamin D, vitamin E and possibly vitamin C. The B vitamins which appear to be most closely related to the health of the adrenals are pantothenic acid, choline, para-amino-benzoic acid (PABA), vitamin B12 and folic acid. Anyone whose meals and snacks contain large amounts of refined carbohydrates is almost bound to be short on these nutrients, for they are simply not present in foods of this kind. And sugars rob the body of B vitamins, since these vitamins are necessary for processing of sugars in the digestive tract. When they are non-existent in foods, they are stolen from body tissues.

Fasting on fruit and vegetable juices is regular therapy at some health clinics—mostly in Europe. The theory here is that by eating nothing except the juices of fresh fruits and vegetables, the "poisons" and wastes in the body will be excreted and, since these are responsible for the illness, the patient is cured. It seems only reasonable to ask why the body's own natural apparatus for excreting waste and poisons should not be adequate to perform this task. It is well known that a diet of wholly natural foods rich in fiber will handle any bodily wastes quite efficiently. Poisons are detoxified by the healthy liver and excreted by way of skin, hair, breath, intestines and kidneys.

So perhaps "juice fasting" as it is called, succeeds because it eliminates from the patients' meals all foods to which he or she is allergic, though, of course, this would not be so with people allergic to one or more of the fruits or vegetables from which the juices are made.

One final word on allergies. An excellent book on the subject appeared a number of years ago which was ignored by practically the entire medical profession: *Goodbye Allergies* by Judge Tom R. Blaine. Judge Blaine was allergic to just about everything that might cause allergy. Treated for low blood sugar (hypoglycemia), he lost all his allergies and they never bothered him again, so long as he remained on the diet which prevents low blood sugar. In the book he explains the diet and the reasons for its success.

It is a diet high in protein, with refined carbohydrates eliminated entirely and even unprocessed foods rich in carbohydrates cut to a minimum. Breakfast must be substantial and contain lots of protein with no quickly absorbable sweets and no caffeine. Other meals the same. Snacks, taken several times a day, must also be high in protein (cheese, meats, eggs, nuts, etc.) Judge Blaine's book is available from The Citadel Press, 120 Enterprise Avenue, Secaucus, N.J. 07094 in hardcover for $6.95; paperback, $2.45. Another paperback on the subject is, *Is Low Blood Sugar Making You a Nutritional Cripple?* by Ruth Adams and Frank Murray. It is published by Larchmont Books, New York City, at $1.75.

CHAPTER 9

Is Your Cartilage
Well Nourished?

CARTILAGE IS THE body tissue that is disordered in arthritis. About 60 percent of cartilage consists of a substance called collagen. Collagen provides elasticity to joints.

The metabolic differences recently identified between normal and osteoarthritic human collagen help explain the nature of the degeneration of cartilage in the joints seen in this disease, reports the National Institutes of Health, November 25, 1973.

This finding, reported by Marcel Nimni, Ph.D., and Kalindi Deskmukh, Ph.D., of the University of Southern California School of Medicine, Los Angeles, offers a clue that may help scientists figure out the cause of the crippling condition. Osteoarthritis, a degenerative disease of the joints, is characterized by cartilage destruction in joints exposed to maximal mechanical stress, especially the weight-bearing joints.

In 1969, Edward J. Miller, Ph.D., and Victor Matukas, D.D.S., Ph.D. (both working at the National Institute of Dental Research at the time), discovered that cartilage collagen differs significantly from skin and bone collagen. The investigators suggested that the particular configuration of cartilage collagen might be essential for the structural integrity of the tissue.

Cartilage, which lines the hip and other joints where the bones meet must withstand tremendous mechanical stress from such normal activities as walking, carrying and running, the NIH reports.

Dr. Miller and Dr. Matukas found that cartilage collagen is assembled from three identical chains and that the chain which he then termed $alpha_1(II)$ differs from the $alpha_1$ chain in skin and bone (subsequently renamed $alpha_1(I)$. Skin and bone collagen contain two $alpha_1(I)$ chains and one $alpha_2$ chain, the NIH says.

In their research, Drs. Nimni and Deskmukh compared the collagen from human osteoarthritic joints with that of normal articular cartilage. The tissue samples were taken during surgery from patients whose arthritic joints were replaced with implants and from non-arthritic patients who required bone surgery.

They published their findings in *Science,* August 24, 1973. Preliminary findings by these same investigators published in *Biochemical and Biophysical Research Communications* suggest that lysosomal enzymes, which are significantly increased in osteoarthritis, may play a major role in the development of such an abnormality.

The National Institute of Dental Research engages in collagen studies because the chemistry of connective tissue protein is important in understanding the physiology of the periodontium (which includes gingiva, two supportive fibers, and bone).

Says *Executive Health* in a fine discussion of *The Arthritis Mystery,* "An early change in osteoarthritic cartilage is softening of the cartilage itself. Later there is partial loss of ground substance.

"Cartilage, of course, just as other body tissues, is continually being torn down and replaced. It is subject to mechanical wear and tear. And it would appear that arthritic changes may result when cartilage cells are unable to properly replace and maintain cartilage after damage even from 'normal' use," says the publication.

The medical dictionary defines cartilage as "gristle, a white semiopaque nonvascular connective tissue." In *The Body Has a Head,* Gustav Eckstein describes the formation of collagen over a wound like this, "Collagen fibers formed. The fissure was crossed and recrossed by the fibers. Dame Nature was at her darning. She was restoring the original fabric."

In his book, *The Healing Factor, Vitamin C Against Disease,* Irwin Stone has this to say about collagen.

"Arthritis, rheumatism and other related conditions are often referred to as the collagen diseases because of the definite involvement of this protein in their genesis and cause... collagen makes up about a third of our body's protein content. It is the deprivation of ascorbic acid (vitamin C), with the consequent synthesis of poor quality collagen or no synthesis at all, which brings on the most distressing bone and joint effects of clinical scurvy (the disease of vitamin C deficiency). There can be no doubt about the intimate association of ascorbic acid and the collagen diseases.

"Rivers in 1965, in a review article on the tissue derangements caused by a lack of ascorbic acid, states, 'Abnormalities in this protein (collagen) are basic to the crippling deformities associated with rheumatic diseases and with a number of congenital connective tissue defects.' Robertson, in studies on induced granuloma tissue of prescorbutic and normal guinea pigs, showed that guinea pigs deprived of ascorbic acid for only 14 days produced tissue containing only 2 to 3 per cent collagen, while the tissues in normal guinea pigs contain 14 to 16 per cent."

Stone then discusses other researches which showed that high quality collagen depends on vitamin C which has a chemical action on some of the amino acids or forms of protein used in manufacturing collagen.

Stone tells us of a researcher who, in 1952, gave intravenous doses of six grams (6,000 milligrams) of vitamin C for acute and chronic rheumatism and got "astonishing" results in some cases. He also got good results in lumbago, sciatica and bronchial asthma.

In 1953 another physician found that 8 to 12 grams of vitamin C along with antibiotics were effective in treating rheumatic fever in several serious cases. In 1955 Dr. W. J. McCormick of Canada gave acute rheumatic fever patients one to 10 grams of vitamin C daily "with a rapid and complete recovery in three to four weeks without cardiac complications."

These excellent results must be related to the essential nature of vitamin C for the formation and repair of the substance collagen, along with, perhaps, the power of vitamin C to cure infections of many kinds.

Says *Executive Health,* the "ground substance of collagen contains polysaccharides which can be manufactured only when vitamin C, vitamin A and manganese are present in adequate amounts." Manganese is a trace mineral which is carefully removed from all our processed and refined carbohydrates—white flour and white sugar. So it seems likely that absence of trace minerals like manganese, as the result of a diet in which refined carbohydrates play a large part, may be one important cause of all the collagen diseases.

"Good healthy collagen is made up of molecules that are chemically cross-linked," says *Executive Health.* "One requirement for the cross-linking is copper." This is another trace mineral also missing from refined foods. Another essential is the B vitamin pyridoxine, which has also been removed when carbohydrate foods are refined, and never replaced.

IS YOUR CARTILAGE WELL NOURISHED?

One treatment for arthritis which almost everybody knows about is cortisone, the powerful hormone that stops the agonizing pain but may produce extremely serious side effects. Scientists believe that aspirin, too, eases pain by persuading the pituitary gland to release another hormone, ACTH, which will cause the adrenal glands to produce their hormones which work like cortisone. These hormones diminish inflammation and the destruction of joint cartilage.

Doctors are relucant to give cortisone over long periods of time these days because of its side effects. Why not, instead, see if we can induce the body to produce its own cortisone? Very many nutrients are involved in this process.

Riboflavin (vitamin B2) helps in inducing the pituitary gland to stimulate the adrenal glands. Riboflavin is not easy to get in most diets these days. It is most abundant in liver and dairy products, along with eggs and wholegrains. Vitamin C, perhaps in large amounts, is needed for the health of the adrenals which should be releasing enough of their hormones to prevent the pain and inflammation of arthritis.

Other vitamins which help out in the production of these essential adrenal hormones are: the B vitamins niacin, pantothenic acid, folic acid, biotin, and pyridoxine (vitamin B6), as well as vitamin A.

Why should adrenal glands need so much attention? Why shouldn't they just go about their normal work of producing hormones without the necessity for large doses of vitamins? One thing that impairs their functioning is stress—some prolonged excessive stress like prolonged worry over the illness of a loved one, the stress of unemployment or financial difficulties.

In many cases—some specialists say in every case—of arthritis or related diseases, the disorder begins after a lot of stress. The mourner just home from the funeral after a long siege of illness, suddenly begins to suffer from joint pains although they were never present before. The adrenal glands protect us from stress. That is their main function. When we overwork them by submitting ourselves to too much stress, they give out. They are exhausted. There is no way for them to cry "Help!" They simply stop functioning effectively in an effort to repair themselves. And aching joints are one of the first indications that the adrenals are exhausted. Too exhausted to produce the hormones that prevent pain and inflammation.

Dr. Roger J. Williams in his excellent book, *Nutrition Against Disease,* has this to say about the collagen diseases, arthritis and related disorders: "While medical education has put a damper on experiments in which the nutrition of arthritics might have been studied and manipulated in an expert fashion, there is excellent reason for thinking that if this were done, sufferers could get real rather than palliative relief. There is even a good possibility that individual arthritics will be able—if they are lucky and make intelligent trials—to hit upon particular nutrients or nutrient combinations which will bring relief.

"... On the basis of reports presently available, the items that certainly need to be considered are niacin (niacinamide), pantothenic acid, riboflavin, vitamin A, vitamin B6, vitamin C, magnesium, calcium, phosphate and other minerals. The objective is to feed *adequately* the cells that are involved in keeping the bones, joints and muscles in healthy condition."

CHAPTER 10

Arthritis and Lead Pollution

A BRILLIANT, hardworking and highly original biochemist was John J. Miller, Ph.D., a former editor in chief of *Chemical Abstracts,* the index to which biologists, chemists and physicians go when they want to look up references to various articles in the thousands of scientific and medical publications.

Dr. Miller was also the originator of the process of combining minerals and vitamins in one capsule without spoilage and the process of chelation of foods, fertilizers and drugs. He was also a pioneer in methods of testing hair to determine the mineral status of an individual.

An article of Dr. Miller's appears in the December, 1976 issue of the *Journal of the International Academy of Preventive Medicine.*

Commenting on arthritis in this article, Dr. Miller said, "I could discuss hour after hour the history of the symptoms of the arthritic syndrome, but briefly I can say that the sad part of the story is that for more than 50 years of presumably intensive research, by private foundations and the United States Government laboratories, everyone concerned is admitting that the cause or causes are unknown, and there are no definite plans for resolving this problem.

"In fact the Surgeon General of the United States advised a large audience of laymen in a meeting in Washington, D.C. that many millions of dollars had been spent on arthritis over the years by the federal government and he was sorry to say that they had given up hope of finding a remedy. His estimate at that time was that 13,500,000 persons in this country were classified as chronic arthritic patients."

Dr. Miller then goes on to say that in 1949 a Dr. Blackburn discovered that a certain enzyme, hyaluronidase, which has been found to be involved in the breakdown of connective tissues and synovial fluids in the body, is "activated" only by the metal lead. The connective tissues of the body are called collagen. The arthritic diseases are called the collagen diseases, because they involve these tissues.

The synovial fluid is the clear fluid resembling the white of a raw egg, which is found in joints, bursa and sheaths of tendons. Joints, bursa (as in bursitis) and tendons (as in tendonitis) are the parts of the body disordered in the arthritic diseases.

Now if, indeed, this particular enzyme has the capacity to break down connective tissues and destroy synovial fluid, it might certainly have something to do with initiating the process of arthritic diseases. But if the only way this enzyme can be activated to do its dirty work is through exposure to the poisonous trace metal lead, then it seems possible, doesn't it, that exposure to lead may have something to do with promoting the breakdown of these tissues that results in arthritis?

Says Dr. Miller, "The conclusion must be that the properties of lead as a spreading factor (that is, breaking down tissues) should be thoroughly investigated not only in connection with arthritis, but with other diseases where the collagen tissues are in similar fashion destroyed."

But, alas, searching through all subsequent medical and scientific literature, as he was easily able to do in his position as editor of *Chemical Abstracts,* Dr. Miller was never able to find a single piece of information regarding this astonishing fact. No other scientist apparently, at least not any working in our country, has ever taken up this matter and considered it in terms of the arthritic diseases. Nor has anyone done research to see if, indeed, exposure to lead can be at least one of the causes of arthritis.

"So," says Dr. Miller, "this disease, that was known to be prevalent among the Egyptians at the time of the Pharoahs, is still the plague of mankind. Yet, it is still an incurable malady requiring pain-killing drugs or hormones too dangerous to use. Many millions of people suffer from arthritis throughout the world today, and hundreds of millions have gone to premature death because of it."

In ancient days people were exposed to lead poisoning without knowing the dangers. Containers for storing food were usually made of lead. If acidic foods or beverages were stored in them (wine, for example) large amounts of lead would leach into the food or drink from the container. Some historians believe that the Roman Empire was destroyed by lead, that lead poisoning from this source rendered the leaders of the Roman Empire so ill and so incapable of guiding the nation that they were easily overcome by their enemies.

Today, in cities around the world, studies are being made of lead poisoning and threats of lead poisoning in homes where old lead-based paint has flaked from the walls. Slum children, cooped up all day inside with nothing much to do, often eat the lead flakes. A recent study involved 27 cities in 23 states. In 85 per cent of them dangerous amounts of flaking lead paint were found. The investigators tested 2,309 children living in these old houses and found that almost 10 per cent have blood levels of lead above what the FDA authorities believe is "safe." One or two of these children had the classic symptoms of lead poisoning. In others those symptoms are possibly still to come. This study was reported in the June 21, 1973 issue of *Medical Tribune*.

In 1973, over protests of the paint industry, the FDA banned the manufacture of high-lead paints. The allowable levels are only 0.5 per cent of lead. However, the Federal Department of Housing and Development has exempted itself from this ban on lead paint in new housing that was under construction at the time. Much of this, of course, would be housing for the children who are now risking lead poisoning in their old tumbledown homes. And almost nothing is done to remove the old lead paint which is the real hazard.

Meanwhile, authorities are finding many children with raised blood levels of lead who do not live in slum houses or eat flaked paint, *Chemical and Engineering News* for February 14, 1972, reports the probable reason: lead in the air of cities from leaded gasoline. This report, which was a letter to the editor signed by the Graduate Class in Environmental Chemistry at Loyola University, points out that measuring just the lead in the air does not give a true picture. When the air pollution stirred up in big city traffic settles to the ground, the dust may contain up to 6 per cent lead by weight—60,000 ppm—far, far more than any allowable levels of this highly toxic substance. Every chemist is taught that lead salts are toxic. Every chemist is aware that tetraethyl lead is added to gasoline. So why have we allowed this situation to develop? the graduate students ask.

The July 21, 1973 issue of *Science News* states that, "A few months ago, the Environmental Protection Agency reported over a fourth of all American children have levels of lead in their bodies that border on toxicity."

Of the 18 tons of lead deposited daily on Los Angeles, most is immobile, apparently accumulating, except for the 4.3-ton dose blown daily into adjacent areas, Dr. J. J. Huntzicker and Dr. S. D. Friedlander of the California Institute of Technology told the 166th national meeting of the American Chemical Society, Chicago, Illinois, August 29, 1973.

Vegetables grown alongside superhighways in our country have been found to contain 50 times more lead than the amount considered tolerable in food. They pick it up from the exhaust of cars and trucks. Says *New Scientist* for December 5, 1963, "Countless people may be regularly swallowing minute amounts but dangerous quantities of poisonous metallic elements. But this is not only because man is busily poisoning his environment, but also because feeding growing populations means huge quantities of food are now being grown or reared on land never before used for the purpose and which may contain harmful substances."

An August 13, 1972 release from the College of Medicine and Dentistry of New Jersey noted that many children chew on bits of newspaper or magazine. Printer's ink contains large amounts of lead. Such children may be getting far too much for their own good. And what happens to the lead when city incinerators burn newspapers and magazines? Well, it floats off into the air and adds to the already heavy burden of lead pollution caused by traffic.

In July, 1972, a Boston health official told the press that a considerable amount of lead may be eroding from the surface of lead water pipes and getting into the drinking water of Boston and possibly other cities. Dr. Dorothy Worth said: "Lead piping is still in wide use throughout the U.S., and anywhere you have lead pipe and corrosive water, you could have lead poisoning."

In several parts of the country airborne lead from industrial plants threatens the health of people living nearby. Dr. Henry Schroeder has stated, "Evidence of a biochemical abnormality in persons exposed to urban air concentrations of lead is beginning to appear. There is little doubt that, at the present rate of pollution, diseases due to lead toxicity will emerge within a few years."

Dr. Robert A. Kehoe of the University of Cincinnati Kettering Laboratories says there is some lead in all food that we eat. He puts the average daily consumption at 0.3 milligrams.

The National Air Pollution Control Administration estimates that 200,000 tons of lead are added to the atmosphere each year and that 95 per cent of this is from automobile exhausts.

Dr. Carl C. Pfeiffer, in his classic book, *Mental and Elemental Nutrients,* says that canned pet food is loaded with lead because of the many organ meats considered unsuitable for human food which are ground into the pet foods. Those most highly nutritious foods, made from liver, are also, often, found to have a high lead content—as high as 7.6 parts per million in beef liver. The copper sulfate sometimes added to the diet of hogs may also leave unwelcome traces of this heavy metal in liver sausage.

For many years evaporated milk has been sold in cans whose soldering contributes traces of lead to the milk inside. Since this is used by many mothers for making baby formulas, many of our children get even more lead from this source, which is added to that picked up by city children playing in traffic-heavy streets and playgrounds nearby. Many hyperactive children have been found to have much more lead in their bodies than they should have.

In the meantime it is noteworthy that one nutrient in which many Americans are deficient is a powerful agent against lead and renders it non-toxic. The nutrient is calcium, an essential mineral. Calcium-deficient animals given water containing lead are found to have bones in which the lead replaced the natural calcium which should be in the bone cells. By giving animals enough calcium, scientists have found they can prevent their digestive tracts from absorbing lead in their food. Calcium protects both water and body tissues from lead contamination. So "hard" water which contains more calcium than "soft" water is protective against lead poisoning.

So far as we can discover, no experiments either with animals or human beings have been done to confirm or disprove the theory that lead in our food, air and water *may* activate a destructive enzyme which *may* destroy collagen tissues and synovial fluid and hence be one precipitating cause of arthritis. We do know that arthritic diseases are on the increase, even among babies.

Why wait until such experiments are done, if, indeed, they ever will be done? Why not check every aspect of daily life in order to remove as much exposure to lead as possible, and then make certain you are getting enough and more than enough calcium, along with vitamin D (from sunshine or fish liver oils) to help you absorb the calcium. Calcium is most abundant in dairy products—milk, cheese and yogurt. It is also available in supplements. There is no indication that the healthy person can get too much calcium, for our bodies have efficient regulatory systems for managing this mineral.

CHAPTER 11

Arthritis and
an Amino Acid

WHAT ONE COULD certainly describe as a "breakthrough" in the study of rheumatoid arthritis occurred in 1971 when the National Institutes of Health announced they had produced great improvement in arthritis patients using enormous doses of an amino acid or form of protein.

In recent years it has been fairly common for researchers to study the effects of large doses of amino acids in treating various conditions of ill health. Amino acids are forms of protein, the building blocks of this basic material from which we are made. The amino acids in food are constructed according to various patterns. Our bodies rearrange these patterns to combine various amino acids to make body protein.

The "breakthrough" mentioned above was performed by an Associate Professor of Medicine at Downstate Medical Center in New York. Dr. Donald A. Gerber, studying rheumatic arthritis, discovered that there appears to be very little histidine in the blood of arthritics. Histidine is one of the 10 amino acids which are essential in food. Others can be manufactured in the body. But essential ones like histidine must be provided in food.

Dr. Gerber found that the blood of arthritics contains

only about one-fourth as much histidine as the blood of healthy people. He began to give a group of arthritis patients large doses of the protein—about six grams a day. Then he gave them various tests for measuring improvement or lack of improvement as time went on. Stiffness and pain as well as range of movement are considered in such tests.

He found that the protein seemed to benefit these patients greatly. Some of them showed improvement with only one gram of histidine daily, others needed as much as six. Nutrition experts do not know why. It all comes under the heading of "biochemical individuality," as Dr. Roger Williams puts it. Each individual is different and has differing nutritional needs.

When Dr. Linus Pauling recommended taking enormous doses of vitamin C to prevent colds, he pointed out that the amount needed may vary from 2.3 grams per day to 9 grams per day. In his book, *Vitamin C and the Common Cold,* Dr. Pauling quotes a practicing physician who believes that getting enough vitamin C right from childhood on may produce an individual "highly resistant to the rheumatoid disease process." This physician has given arthritics as much as 25 to 50 grams of vitamin C daily and has never produced any unpleasant side effects. Dr. Irwin Stone, author of *The Healing Factor, Vitamin C Against Disease,* says that vitamin C "is probably the least toxic of any known substance of comparable physiologic activity."

If it is true that individual requirements for vitamins and minerals can vary by these huge amounts, isn't it also quite possible that individuals vary in their need for various forms of protein, or amino acids? Such excessive need might be determined by one's heredity, which might help to explain why many of these degenerative diseases "run in families."

ARTHRITIS

It seems certain that this must be the determining factor in Dr. Gerber's treatment. When he finds the correct level of the amino acid histidine for each patient and the individual continues to take that amount, it seems possible that this debilitating and extremely painful disease may be conquered. Doctors have almost no other remedy for arthritis, except those massive doses of aspirin year after year to deaden the pain. Aspirin taken in such quantities may produce very unpleasant side effects.

As usual with new research of this kind, the National Institutes of Health in Washington has warned that the work is only beginning and that Dr. Gerber must carry out many more experiments to determine just how the amino acid works and why it produces varying results in different people.

There is also the possibility that massive doses of an amino acid, taken alone for many years or for life, may have disturbing side effects, in some people at least. The amino acid in food, in much smaller amounts, well balanced with all the other amino acids, along with starch, vitamins, minerals and everything else that is in food, cannot harm you unless you happen to have been born with an inability to deal with this one amino acid. This would probably have been evident at birth.

But we do not apparently have enough information on long-term use of histidine to guarantee its safety, even if it were available at the drug store or a health food store. It is our hope that many physicians, treating arthritis patients, will get in touch with Dr. Gerber, ask how his work is going and whether it seems advisable for other physicians to use this amino acid as a weapon against arthritis.

The best we lay people can do, if we would prevent arthritis or possibly relieve early symptoms of this disease, is to eat lots of those foods in which histidine is plentiful. In fact, it might be a good idea to restrict our foods mostly to those in which there is plenty of histidine, along with fruits and vegetables to supply missing nutrients like vitamins A and C.

These are the foods in which histidine is most plentiful: whole eggs, whole milk, liver, meat, corn germ, fish, wheat germ, soybean meal, brown rice, whole wheat, wheat gluten, brewers yeast, peanut flour and other foods in the seed group like dried peas and beans and soy beans. The histidine content of wheat gluten is so high that we might suggest the use of gluten bread for arthritics. This is usually available at health food stores.

There is no way of knowing whether an arthritic can get enough histidine just by using these foods every day, especially since people vary so much in their need for this amino acid. Since these are all excellent foods, nutritionally speaking, anyone using them would undoubtedly improve so far as health is concerned, whether or not the arthritis improves. So there is no reason not to try.

CHAPTER 12

Pyridoxine for Early Arthritis Symptoms

THE B VITAMIN PYRIDOXINE (vitamin B6) is known to be essential for many body functions, including the processes by which our bodies break down and utilize fats, proteins and carbohydrates, which are the main elements in our daily foods.

Recent investigations have shown that many conditions of ill health seem to respond almost magically to large doses of pyridoxine taken over long periods of time. Arthritis (or rheumatism) seems to be one of these, according to Dr. John Ellis, a Texas physician who has specialized in the use of pyridoxine for many mysterious conditions that would yield to no other therapy.

Dr. Ellis began his use of vitamin B6 when he noticed that patients complained of trouble with their hands. There is a numbness or tingling in hands and fingers. The little finger may be the first to be involved. The patient may complain that his hands "go to sleep" when he is in bed at night. Fingers may become stiff so that it is almost impossible to "make a fist." There is pain in the joints and the grip becomes so weak that things are easily dropped.

The hands may swell, then, so that rings become too tight. At night an entire arm may appear to be paralyzed, so that the other arm must be used to shake it "awake." The sense of touch may be affected so that, with eyes closed, the patient cannot tell the difference in texture between glass and rough wood. "Charley horse" or leg cramps may be very troublesome at night, while the patient vainly tries to massage the cramping leg back to some degree of comfort.

Little knots or bumps may appear at the side of fingers. Doctors call these *Heberden's Nodes*. Then arms and shoulders may be affected. Pain may be located in the shoulder, below it or in the arm between the shoulder and elbow. Questioned about his condition, the patient will say, "I have rheumatism."

And Dr. Ellis, in a chapter in the massive book, *A Physician's Handbook on Orthomolecular Medicine,* says, about this condition, "The people studied in Northeast Texas, and there were hundreds, perhaps thousands that I saw, did have rheumatism and they exhibited spectacular response to vitamin B_6 given 50 milligrams daily by mouth.... There are dozens of patients in Northeast Texas who have taken pyridoxine, 50 milligrams daily for eight years, and there are thousands who have taken pyridoxine, 50 milligrams daily for the last four years."

He goes on to say, "Motion pictures taken before and after treatment with pyridoxine have objective proof that vitamin B6 reduced swelling in hands and fingers, improved range of finger flexion, improved speed of finger flexion, improved coordination of finger movement, prevented transitory nocturnal arm paralysis, and halted nighttime leg cramps and muscle spasms. Subjectively, after six weeks of therapy, there was improvement of sensation and perception in finger tips, and there was elimination of numbness and tingling in hands and fingers.

Shoulder pain was reduced or eliminated, and shoulder and arm function was improved. Finger joints that had been tender and painful before treatment were substantially improved after six weeks of therapy with pyridoxine."

Dr. Ellis goes on to relate his experiences giving pyridoxine in doses up to 300 milligrams to pregnant women and reducing dramatically the painful swelling in their hands and feet—and this without any reduction of salt in their diets and without diuretics or "water pills." Pyridoxine has been found to be seriously deficient in many women on The Pill. Is it possible that all troubles with edema or swelling of hands and feet in pregnant women may be caused simply by lack of vitamin B6?

"Onset of the disease syndrome known as rheumatism was gradual (among his patients)," says Dr. Ellis. "There was edema of hands and fingers long before there was experience of pain and stiffness in shoulders. Occasionally there was a rather sudden onset of signs and symptoms that has been alluded to as the 'shoulder-hand-syndrome.' The long-standing cases were more difficult to relieve, and ordinarily the older aged people had less response to pyridoxine. There was no doubt, however, that patients with the 'shoulder-hand-syndrome' exhibited improvement of hand function, reduction of edema (swelling) and moderate relief of pain in shoulders when pyridoxine was given 50 to 100 milligrams daily for six weeks. Reduction of edema and improvement in hand function could be observed within one week of initiation of treatment."

Dr. Ellis is quick to point out that other nutrients are important too. Pyridoxine is not a "miracle drug" that can guarantee instant relief of pain and swelling if an atrocious diet is eaten and all the other vitamins and minerals are ignored. Dr. Ellis suggests wheat germ as an excellent source of pyridoxine. Brewers yeast, too, is a good source, though not so tasty, hence a bit more difficult to work into one's diet. Leafy vegetables—the dark green ones like spinach and watercress, turnip greens and broccoli—are also good sources of vitamin B6, as well as other B vitamins and many minerals.

Most of all, one should avoid all those foods from which the pyridoxine and most other nutrients have been removed, for these foods present your body with a dilemma that it cannot solve and remain healthy. The foods we mean are white sugar and white flour and every food made from them. They contain relatively huge amounts of carbohydrates from which practically all of the B vitamins, the minerals and trace minerals have been removed in the refining process. These B vitamins, minerals and trace minerals are absolutely essential for your body to use carbohydrates healthfully.

When they are lacking—and they are lacking in the average American diet loaded with sugar and white bread—things are bound to go wrong, healthwise. Arthritis or rheumatism is one of the penalties we pay for not recognizing this fact and for continuing to buy and eat these staple and popular foods.

You can feel perfectly safe in taking large amounts of pyridoxine. Like all other B vitamins, it is water soluble. Whatever is not used is rather quickly excreted. It is not stored in the body tissues to any great extent. By the same token, you should take all of the B vitamins, including pyridoxine, frequently. Don't think a few hundred milligrams once a week or once a month will accomplish anything. You need these nutrients every day. If you happen to be one of those individuals who need large amounts of pyridoxine or other B vitamins, then you need large amounts every day, not just occasionally when you remember to take them.

Dr. Ellis feels that only one caution is necessary in regard to vitamin B6. There is some evidence, he says, that pyridoxine "has something to do with histamine production and very likely it increases production or action of stomach secretions. At any rate, people who have stomach ulcers should be under treatment before beginning use of vitamin B6."

For women on The Pill, it is necessary to take pyridoxine every day along with the many other nutrients that this hormone medication destroys in the body. The Pill is creating a condition of pregnancy in the woman's body every month. All the extraordinary measures the body calls into play to conduct a successful pregnancy are called upon. Then The Pill is stopped for a period of menstruation, and the body's elaborate preparations for pregnancy are stalled. The next month the same cycle takes place. No wonder essential nutrients are wasted and disappear from the body, creating deficiencies whose full destructive power may not be demonstrated for years.

Pyridoxine is one of these nutrients. It also seems to be deficient in people who are just beginning to notice the advance of arthritis symptoms. Replacing it by taking a daily supplement is only common sense. Since no one knows how much any individual may need of this B vitamin, it's best to be safe rather than sorry. Taking more of the B vitamins than you may need is insurance, the best kind of health insurance there is.

CHAPTER 13

Vitamin B3
and Arthritis

A FASCINATING, long out of print book—published in Brattleboro, Vermont in 1949—described how a doctor used niacinamide, the amide form of the B vitamin niacin or vitamin B3, to treat many patients suffering from arthritis. The doctor was William Kaufman, Ph.D., M.D., and the name of his book was *The Common Form of Joint Dysfunction: Its Incidence and Treatment*. Here are some case histories.

1. A 60-year-old accountant came to Dr. Kaufman with severe joint dysfunction or arthritis. He was given 160 milligrams of vitamin B3 every two hours for eight doses daily (1,200 milligrams in 24 hours). In 315 days of such therapy his arthritis improved from a rating of "severe" to "slight."

2. A 30-year-old woman came into Dr. Kaufman's office complaining of moderate arthritis, transient low back pain, right shoulder discomfort, persistent stiffness of joints. She had had a "nervous breakdown" several years earlier when her husband died. She had had "the usual" menopause symptoms. She was given 150 milligrams of niacinamide to take every three hours for six daily doses. Within one month her joint troubles had greatly improved. On the advice of a

friend, she decided to take less of the B vitamin. Her condition worsened. When she went back to the original dose, she improved.

3. A 61-year-old engineer came to Dr. Kaufman's office with severe persistent headaches, from which he could get no relief. In the past two years the headaches had become much worse. His joints grated, especially in the neck. He was stiff in the morning when first awake, also when the weather was bad. His shoulders had been painful with intermittent stiffness and pain in finger joints. He was given the B vitamin in doses of 160 milligrams at regular intervals to equal 975 milligrams per day. His headaches improved gradually. Within 190 days his arthritic condition improved from "severe" to "slight." He was also given large doses of vitamin C, along with smaller doses of riboflavin (vitamin B2) and thiamine (vitamin B1).

4. A 45-year-old attorney came to Dr. Kaufman's office with severe joint dysfunction. He was given 1,800 milligrams of niacinamide every 24 hours, along with other B vitamins and vitamin C. Within 178 days of therapy, his condition was greatly improved.

Dr. Kaufman, determined to conquer arthritis for at least some of his patients, developed elaborate devices for measuring what he called "joint dysfunction"—that is, anything which impaired the patient's ability to move about—any dysfunction of arms, legs, wrists, back and so on. By measuring the patient's grasp, reach and other extensions of joints, he was able to classify their ailment according to the numbers on the mechanism he had invented. As time went on, the same patient was asked to perform the same motions, so that improvement or lack of it could be measured and noted. Dr. Kaufman was not content merely to ask the patient, "How are your joints today?" He could physically measure any improvement or lack of improvement.

VITAMIN B3 AND ARTHRITIS

The case histories in this book are almost unbelievable, especially in view of the fact that it was written almost 30 years ago, when vitamins were almost never spoken of in terms of preventive medicine and when the idea of using vitamins in massive doses had not even been considered by most researchers or physicians. Dr. Kaufman was an innovator—many years ahead of his time.

Also of interest is the fact that he made no other changes in his patients' lives except for the vitamins he gave them. There is no mention throughout the book of revising their diets, asking them to exercise more or make any other changes in their way of life. So the record appears to be just a record mostly of what one vitamin—niacinamide—can do to improve the condition of patients with painful stiff joints. It seems to us that far better or perhaps quicker results might have occurred had the patients been placed on diets in which all refined carbohydrates were restricted, and emphasis was laid on high protein foods and whole, unprocessed foods. But Dr. Kaufman confined his treatment to vitamins alone.

He did not use just niacinamide. In most cases he also gave quite large doses of vitamin C, thiamine (B1), pyridoxine (B6) and riboflavin (B2). He tailored the dosage of niacinamide according to the individual patient's needs. If there appeared to be little or no improvement, he increased the dosage. If improvement appeared to have stopped at a "plateau," he increased the dosage. He cautioned his patients to continue with the recommended dosage even if they became discouraged with slow progress. Improvement with this completely harmless therapy appears to take quite a long time, although in several cases described in the book almost miraculous improvement occurred in a matter of months in people who had suffered for years from arthritis.

Dr. Kaufman mentions several things which complicate

treatment. These are things we might have neglected to notice in ourselves. But a very detailed history sometimes turned up significant items in regard to the possible causes of the complaint.

Sometimes it was allergy. Some of his patients knew they were allergic to certain foods: wheat, chocolate, eggs, etc. When they carefully avoided these foods, their improvement was assured. If they transgressed and ate even small amounts of the offending foods, their condition invariably worsened.

Another drawback to continued improvement usually had to do with repetitive work done every day by the patient in an uncomfortable or awkward position. This is almost bound to create joint problems which will not yield to any treatment. Anyone working with tools or machinery, twisting a foot around the leg of a chair while sitting, holding the phone in an awkward position for long conversation, maintaining poor posture year after year, wearing uncomfortable shoes or high heels, or socks that are too short. Dr. Kaufman describes a woman whose joint pains occurred only on certain days. It developed that these were the days when she ironed. She habitually held the iron in a tight grip and pressed hard on the ironing board, as well as pulling tightly on the object she was ironing. Correcting these improper methods of work greatly alleviated her joint pains.

Another complicating factor in arthritis, says Dr. Kaufman, is sodium retention. Many women complain of this several days before their menstrual period: bloating, weight gain, irritability, discomfort, insomnia caused by the body retaining sodium or salt. Some people appear to retain salt more readily than others. And, of course, some people eat far more salt than others. We believe that everyone should use as little salt as possible in cooking— just enough to add a bit of flavor to extremely bland foods.

And no salt should be added at the table.

Dr. Kaufman believed there is a kind of psychosomatic arthritis. People living under constant stress or under unbearable conditions which seemingly cannot be changed may develop joint symptoms which are not actually physical but are brought about by life circumstances, whether they are imagined or real.

Dr. Kaufman's conclusions are these: "During the first month of adequate therapy with niacinamide (alone or in combination with other vitamins), a patient with joint dysfunction (with or without rheumatic or hypertrophic arthritis) will have a rise in the Joint Range Index of at least 6-12 points, and thereafter will have a rise of at least one-half to 1 point per month of adequate niacinamide therapy, provided he eats the average American diet containing adequate calories and sufficient protein, and provided he does not mechanically injure his joints excessively. This improvement in joint mobility occurs regardless of the age or sex of the patient and regardless of whatever other health problems he may have. Subsequently, with continuously adequate niacinamide therapy, the Joint Range Index of 96-100 (no joint dysfunction) is reached and maintenance doses of niacinamide are required to keep the Index at this level." The only exception to this rule, he says, is the patient whose joints are ankylosed—that is, immovably fixed in one position. Such patients cannot ever achieve perfect range of movement, says Dr. Kaufman.

The patient must go on taking niacinamide. If he stops, the symptoms gradually recur. If, after he has achieved the best possible dosage for him, he reduces the dosage, he will regress to whatever degree of improvement such a dosage can produce for him individually. Dr. Kaufman says his patients derive other benefits from the vitamin treatment. Digestive complaints may disappear. They may feel more alert, more vigorous. They may tire less easily. Liver tenderness and enlargement may disappear. Muscle strength seems to improve.

"In the last stages of rheumatic arthritis there may be so much retrogressive tissue alteration in non-articular as well as articular tissue, that complete functional and structural recovery may not be possible, even with prolonged niacinamide therapy," says Dr. Kaufman. He tells us, too, that he does not know why or how niacinamide acts to improve the condition of painful, stiff joints. He hopes that more research will be done on this. He does believe, however, that the "evolution of the common form of joint dysfunction can be prevented by adequate niacinamide supplementation of an adequate diet throughout the lifetime of an individual."

Other investigations in earlier years have turned up much valuable evidence that vitamin C is essential, in large amounts, to prevent and treat arthritis. Indeed, there seems to be great similarity between the joint symptoms of scurvy, the disease of vitamin C deficiency, and arthritis. In each case the collagen is disordered. This is the substance of which we are made, especially joints. Vitamin C is essential for the manufacture of collagen. In its absence, as in scurvy, collagen simply wastes away until the poor scurvy victim cannot walk or endure the pain of moving his joints. Is it not possible that modern arthritis may be caused in part at least by all the demands made on our vitamin C stores by all the poisons in our environment, along with the fact that many of us simply don't get enough vitamin C to meet our needs?

Practically all researchers on arthritis stress the need for an adequate diet with plenty of protein and elimination of sugar and all foods that contain it. Past researchers have turned up the fact that arthritics tend to eat lots of sugar. Many are victims of low blood sugar which is corrected by a diet in which sugar is eliminated and protein is stressed.

VITAMIN B3 AND ARTHRITIS

Early investigations turned up the fact that children who developed rheumatic heart conditions did not like or did not eat eggs when they were young. Perhaps the bounty of high quality protein, plus the vitamins and minerals of eggs are far more important than we know in preventing the aches and disability of arthritis.

We do not know why Dr. Kaufman's fine, well-documented book was not followed up by many more investigations of the power of the B vitamin niacinamide against arthritis. Perhaps some modern physician may take up the fight where Dr. Kaufman left off. We hope so. Meanwhile, there seems to be no reason not to apply his findings in your own life. He reported absolutely no harmful side effects from these very large doses of vitamin B3. This vitamin is also being used in very large doses in treating schizophrenia, with almost no reports of side effects in doses much larger than those used by Dr. Kaufman.

As we reported earlier, Dr. Kaufman's book is out of print. Several years ago a few copies were available at $35 each. This is a book for physicians, not laymen; a layman would have difficulty reading through the medical jargon. Physicians and other professionals can contact Mrs. Charlotte Kaufman, 540 Brooklawn Avenue, Bridgeport, Conn. 06604 as to whether or not any of the books are left or whether she has had it reprinted.

CHAPTER 14

Arthritis and Pantothenic Acid

AFTER THOUSANDS OF years of investigation and treatment, medical men and scientists are still baffled by the disease called arthritis. They are still unable to pinpoint any exact and always-present cause, still helpless to do much more than prescribe physical therapy and painkillers. However, new methods of working in laboratories, new ways of delving into the mysteries of nutrition are turning up startling new facts in regard to this ancient disorder.

An investigation of an important B vitamin in relation to rheumatoid arthritis is reported in *The Lancet* for October 26, 1963. Two London doctors tested the amount of pantothenic acid in the blood of various persons, including some arthritics. They found that, for some reason, the blood of people with arthritis contains considerably less of this B vitamin than that of healthy people. They also found that the lower the amount of pantothenic acid in the blood, the more severe were the symptoms of arthritis. Patients whose blood levels were lowest of all were bedridden and badly crippled!

Interestingly enough, they also found that vegetarians (not vegans—but people who eat milk and eggs) had, generally speaking, higher levels of pantothenic acid than people who consume meat every day in a well-balanced diet.

Is it possible that the rheumatic condition of these people might be due, even partly, to lack of pantothenic acid? The researchers thought they might find some answer to this question by injecting the B vitamin into a group of 20 arthritic patients every day. After seven days of injections the patients' symptoms improved and their blood levels of pantothenic acid rose. There was no further improvement, however, even though the injections were continued for another three weeks. As soon as the injections stopped, the blood levels of the vitamin dropped again.

So, as the authors say, it seems there is some other essential factor or factors which govern the body's use of pantothenic acid and its levels in the blood. Its nature is not known.

We do know, however, that royal jelly, the food fed to larval bees to produce queens, is the richest natural source of pantothenic acid. So the doctors injected royal jelly into a group of arthritic patients every day for a month. There was no change in their condition. When they injected both royal jelly and the B vitamin some of the patients improved and their joints moved more easily. But the improvement was not permanent. However, when these same injections were given to arthritic vegetarians, symptoms disappeared rapidly and, in nine patients at least, the symptoms did not return.

Some of the patients suffered from the injections and others did not improve, say the doctors. They plan to continue their research.

From a Japanese journal, the *Tohoku Journal of Experimental Medicine* for November 25, 1961, we find that a survey of 200 Japanese showed that levels of pantothenic acid declined in the blood from the age of 30 on. We think of arthritis as a disease of middle and old age.

In the *Journal of Nutrition* for December 1961, we find that those whose requirements for pantothenic acid are very high may need much more of this B vitamin than relatives or friends need.

This is true, we know, of other vitamins as well. The daily requirement for this vitamin is believed to be about 10 to 15 milligrams, although this is not official. Since the vitamin is present in many common foods, it is generally assumed among nutritionists that no one in the United States could ever become deficient in it.

There is one very important expert who does not agree—the man who discovered pantothenic acid in his laboratory at the University of Texas—Dr. Roger J. Williams. He named the vitamin pantothenic from the Greek word meaning "from everywhere" because it seemed to be present in everything. But he says, in his book, *Nutrition in a Nutshell,* "Whether or not human beings are subject to pantothenic acid deficiency depends on how their needs compare quantitatively with the available supply. Wide distribution without regard to the quantities has nothing whatever to do with the question of human deficiencies. The quantitative aspects of nutrition are all important."

In other words, it does not matter how much pantothenic acid there is in the food you individually eat. If you happen to need far more than that, you are going to be deficient in this important vitamin. Dr. Williams says that, since human milk contains about 18 times more pantothenic acid than thiamine (vitamin B1), it would seem that we need about 18 times more in our everyday meals. Although pantothenic acid is not destroyed to any extent in cooking, as some vitamins are, dry heat is very destructive of this vitamin. So toasting bread causes a loss of pantothenic acid.

Based on the *Lancet* article, can we say with firmness

that pantothenic acid and/or royal jelly have been proved to be of benefit in the treatment or prevention of rheumatoid arthritis? No, we cannot. We must wait for further research. Perhaps scientists will some day find the missing link—the substance that works with the B vitamin to keep blood levels high and joints supple. Perhaps they may soon find out a great deal more about individual requirements for the vitamins—why some of us need so much more of the vitamins than others and how all the

Pantothenic Acid in Foods—
Milligrams per serving
It is recommended that you get
10–15 milligrams per day

Bananas	0.3	Oysters	0.5
Beans, dried lima	0.8	Peaches	0.1
Beef brain	2.1 to 2.9	Peas, fresh	0.6 to 1
Beef heart	2.1 to 2.9	Peanuts	2.5
Beef kidney	3.4	Pork, bacon	0.2 to 0.9
Beef liver	5.7 to 8.2	Pork, ham	0.3 to 0.6
Beef muscle	1.1	Pork, kidney	3.1
Bread, whole wheat	0.5	Pork, liver	5.9 to 7.3
Broccoli	1.4	Pork, muscle	0.4 to 1.5
Cauliflower	0.9	Potatoes, white	0.4 to 0.6
Cheese	0.5 to 0.9	Potatoes, sweet	0.9
Chicken	0.5 to 0.9	Salmon	0.6 to 1
Eggs	2.7	Soybeans	1.8
Lamb	0.6	Tomatoes	0.3
Lamb kidney	4.3	Wheat, whole	1.3
Milk, whole	0.6	Wheat germ	2
Mushrooms	1.7	Wheat bran	2.4
Oranges	0.3		

vitamins are related to our total health. Perhaps they will uncover the reason why vegetarians have higher blood levels of this vitamin than the rest of us.

In the October 7, 1966 issue of *Medical World News,* three London researchers relate arthritis to a lack of pantothenic acid in the blood. They tested the blood of normal people and arthritics for its pantothenic acid content. In a healthy person they found that the level is about 107 micrograms in a given measure, whereas in arthritics it averages only about 68.7 micrograms. In fact, they found that any patient with less than 95 micrograms showed some symptoms of arthritis. And the lower the level of the B vitamin, the more severe the symptoms.

In other tests, they found that several other substances which are closely involved with pantothenic acid in digestion were also at abnormal levels in arthritics. They injected into their patients these substances that were missing. They gave daily injections of pantothenic acid for one month. There were no results. No improvement.

But the doctors were not so easily discouraged. They were sure some other substance must be missing, too. "We had one clue as to what this might be," said one of the scientists. "The richest natural source of pantothenic acid is royal jelly, the larval food of the queen bee. Royal jelly is also the richest source of another substance, with the tongue twisting name of 10-hydroxy-delta 2-decenoic acid."

The physicians injected pantothenic acid along with royal jelly into 20 of their rheumatoid arthritis patients. In 14 there was improvement in their symptoms. They were able to move more readily and other symptoms characteristic of the disease disappeared, so long as the patients continued to take the injections. Later, the doctors found a cheaper substitute for the very expensive and rare substance in royal jelly. And they found they could get results by giving this substance, along with pantothenic acid, by mouth rather than by injection.

Working with osteoarthritic patients, they added a substance called cysteine to the pantothenic acid and got excellent results with these patients, too. How much did they give? They had no guidelines to go by. So they experimented until they found the dosage that produced results.

Sometimes they were slow in coming. There seems to be no improvement for the first four to eight weeks. But, says one of the doctors, "Just when the patient is deciding that the cure is no good, the symptoms disappear overnight." The treatment must be maintained indefinitely or the symptoms return. But this leaves the arthritic in no worse condition than the diabetic who must take insulin indefinitely. If he can prevent the agonizing symptoms of this extremely painful disease, he would surely be willing to swallow a few pills every day from now on.

Dr. Roger Williams tells the story of the London research discussed in *The Lancet* article in his fine book, *Nutrition Against Disease*. Dr. E. C. Barton-Wright and his colleagues were investigating pantothenic acid when they decided to try it on arthritics.

"What would have happened," asks Dr. Williams, "if the patients in London had also received an abundance of niacinamide (vitamin B3) and other essentials? We do not know. But regardless of what else the ailing cells may need, it appears likely that pantothenic acid is one of the nutritional elements that is often in short supply."

He mentions pyridoxine (vitamin B6), folic acid, another B vitamin, vitamin A and many minerals including calcium and magnesium as being probably also deficient in arthritic conditions.

In other chapters, we related the importance of vitamin C to the health of the adrenal glands, the support of our bodies in times of stress, and to the health of collagen, that biological "glue" which literally holds our bodies together.

All of these nutrients are undoubtedly involved in the health of joints which are disordered in rheumatoid arthritis and osteoarthritis. As Dr. Williams says, "until a more promising alternative appears, I shall continue to invoke the motto, 'When in doubt, try nutrition first!'"

Meanwhile, it is wise to guarantee as much pantothenic acid in your diet as possible, just in case you are one of the people whose requirement is high. The chart shows the pantothenic acid content of some common foods, in terms of 100 grams, which is an average serving. Why not list everything you ate today, then list its pantothenic acid content and total the amount?

A day's menu of an orange and two eggs for breakfast, a cheese sandwich on whole wheat bread for lunch, and a dinner of roast beef, potatoes and a vegetable, with, say, three cups of milk and three more slices of whole grain bread during the day would give you less than 12 milligrams of pantothenic acid.

As you can see from the chart, many of the foods which health-conscious people know are packed with nutrition are the same foods in which pantothenic acid is abundant. Let's eat more of them.

CHAPTER 15

Vitamin D, Vitamin E and Arthritis

THE *British Medical Journal* for November 23, 1974 reported on results of a study which showed that elderly women who have arthritis and associated bone fractures are getting far too little vitamin D in their meals. This deficiency plays an important role in the frequency of bone fractures in these elderly people who have longstanding arthritis. Vitamin D is almost entirely lacking in food. There is some in egg yolk and some fish products like mackerel, tuna and sardines.

In most localities milk is irradiated to produce vitamin D. But we are apparently meant to get our vitamin D from the sunlight falling on our skins. A fatty substance in the skin converts the sunlight into vitamin D. But old folks, especially in a rainy country like England, surely do not get much vitamin D on their skins, especially in winter.

Arthritics of all ages have trouble getting out, so one would assume they are bound to lack the "sunshine vitamin" unless they make special efforts to get it in food, milk and food supplements made from fish liver oil.

According to two Japanese physicians, vitamin E gives

valuable assistance to patients who are being treated with hormones, sometimes called "steroids." These powerful drugs, which alleviate symptoms of pain and swelling also produce such extremely serious side effects that often they must be discontinued. But when vitamin E in quite large doses is given with them, side effects are eliminated and eventually the doses of the powerful drugs can be reduced or stopped.

The two Kyoto Medical College professors used from 150 to 600 milligrams of alpha-tocopherol (vitamin E) daily. They tell the story of one 29-year-old housewife who had rheumatism of the elbows, arms, fingers and legs. Her condition was deteriorating with very high doses of the steroids. And when the doctors tried to reduce the dosage, she returned to the clinic, barely able to walk.

At this point they gave her vitamin E along with the drugs. Seven months later she was discharged on a very small dose of the drug—plus vitamin E. At present, they say, she is "progressing." "She is able to enjoy folk dancing and bicycle riding." That certainly sounds like real progress in a patient who had not been able to walk a few months previously.

The Japanese doctors also reported that other conditions related to blood vessels appear to be gradually improved when vitamin E is given. The vitamin appears to stimulate the circulation in the feet, legs and hands, they say. Furthermore, the vitamin increases the flow of blood in both arteries and veins. Rheumatic patients report that they lose the "cold feeling" in their legs when they are on high doses of vitamin E. The vitamin seems to prevent blood vessels from becoming fragile and to increase the resistance in the walls of the tiny capillaries—the smallest of the blood vessels.

The two Japanese physicians discovered these properties of vitamin E when they treated a patient whose hand had been crushed beneath a great weight. Six months later a circulatory disturbance developed and the fingers began to turn blue and become very painful. The doctors gave large doses of vitamin E. After four months there was great improvement. Then they decided to try vitamin E on their rheumatic patients with the excellent results reported above.

It has been known for a long time that vitamin E is a powerful prop for failing circulatory systems. There are hundreds of reports in medical literature indicating that heart conditions and many other circulatory conditions improve on large doses of vitamin E. Now the Japanese researchers tell us that they have found still more uses for the vitamin, in large doses. They believe it may be effective in preventing the bone softening and the frequent bone fractures that often accompany the use of the steroid drugs.

Now what does all this mean, in terms of healthy people who just want to maintain their daily health? Well, a vitamin which strenghtens walls of blood vessels and increases the flow of blood in both arteries and veins is surely a powerful weapon against both stroke and heart attacks. A vitamin which will prevent small blood vessels from breaking can surely prevent hemorrhages of small vessels in the brain and elsewhere.

A vitamin which can restore the feeling of warmth to limbs so damaged they feel cold most of the time is certainly a valuable asset for everyone who suffers from "poor circulation." A vitamin which stimulates glands is of inestimable value to all of us, for glands determine the healthful functioning of our entire body apparatus. If these glands are sluggish or not doing their work, any and all body mechanisms can easily get out of running order.

The information reported above was contained in an address before the Japanese Rheumatism Society. It was reported in this country in *Medical World News* for July 1,

1966. The editor of the magazine at the time was Morris Fishbein, for many years editor of the *Journal of the American Medical Association*.

In far corners of the world, other researchers are working with vitamin E and uncovering near-miracles which this vitamin can perform. It seems to be involved chiefly with the important job of supplying oxygen to cells. In many disorders, especially those of circulation, the body cannot seem to get enough oxygen, which is essential for good health. Somehow—no one knows how—vitamin E seems to allow cells to get along healthfully without too much oxygen. This may be one way vitamin E works its near-miracles.

Best food sources of vitamin E are wheat germ, whole grain cereals, liver, legumes like peas, beans and soybeans and the salad oils—richest sources of all. Of these, wheat germ oil and soybean oil contain the most vitamin E. You can also buy it in capsules in highly concentrated form.

CHAPTER 16

Trace Minerals in Rheumatoid Arthritis

RHEUMATOID ARTHRITIS IS a disease whose origin is mysterious, whose comings and goings are even more mysterious and unexpected, whose symptoms are agonizing and whose final "cure" may come about apparently through no effort of the patient or the physician or, on the other hand, after years of experimenting with every medical therapy and even all the "quack" remedies.

There seems to be some significance in the relationship of various trace minerals in the body of the arthritic. Here is evidence from medical and scientific journals seeming to indicate that there may be powerful forces at work to disorder the body's use of trace minerals in arthritis, and some evidence that the deficiency in certain trace minerals may be important to the cause of this disease.

In his book, *Trace Elements in Human and Animal Nutrition,* Dr. E. J. Underwood discusses an apparent relationship between the trace mineral manganese and this painful condition. He says that several investigators have found that there are elevated levels of manganese in the red blood cells of arthritis patients although there is no such change in the plasma or liquid part of the blood.

In this investigation whole blood of healthy volunteers contained an average of 9.84 micrograms of manganese per liter, whereas that of arthritics contained 14.99 micrograms. The red blood cells of the healthy individuals contained about 23 micrograms and those of the arthritics about 34 micrograms. This seems to indicate a slow turnover of this trace mineral in the blood of arthritics.

Says Dr. Underwood, the daily intake of manganese will vary greatly with the foods eaten, and especially with the amounts of refined carbohydrates, green leafy vegetables and tea that are eaten. It seems that tea contains considerable manganese. Manganese is almost entirely removed from grain when it is made into white flour. Whole-grain cereal products may contain as much as 91 parts per million of manganese, while nuts contain about 42 ppm, dried beans and other legumes about 28 ppm and green leafy vegetables up to 13 ppm.

Even very large amounts of manganese appear to be non-toxic. As much as 820 ppm in food and supplements produces no bad effect on animals. Some time ago (December 29, 1962), *The Lancet* reported on an astonishing incident which took place in South Africa. A man in a diabetic coma was brought in with blood sugar at fantastically high levels. When he became conscious, he told doctors that he usually controlled the wild swings from high to low blood sugar by drinking alfalfa tea, an old folk remedy. The doctors allowed his blood sugar to rise again to dangerous levels, then told him to brew and drink his alfalfa tea. He did. Blood sugar declined to normal levels almost at once.

A check on the trace minerals in alfalfa disclosed that it contains considerable manganese. The doctors gave their diabetic patient a dose of manganese and his blood sugar remained normal as long as the dosage was continued. This suggests that perhaps the alleviation of arthritis reported by many patients who drink alfalfa tea may have a lot to do with its manganese content.

The effects of gold injections on arthritis have been known for many years. They are helpful, it seems, but too often patients have gotten too much gold and suffered from poisoning. A new way of injecting the gold appears to show promise. California scientists measured the amount of gold already in the patients' blood. They found that different individuals used the gold at different rates, which doesn't seem very surprising. So, adjusting the amount of gold in the injections to keep the blood level consistent all the time seems to solve the problem of getting too much. Some patients get much more than others and apparently need more than others. Just by adjusting the dose, doctors have found that gold treatment can be much less risky.

The processes by which gold enhances the body's defenses against arthritis are complicated. If, as some researchers believe, arthritis is caused by an as yet unknown virus, the body's defense against such a virus would consist of protective blood cells, plus antibodies, all of which are swallowed up by the body cell which contains small sacs called lysosomes, which contain enzymes that digest or dissolve the invading particles.

It is theorized that, in arthritis, the protectors may not be able to call up the usual defenders against the invading enemy. As these "confused" substances enter into the cell, it becomes overly full and emits powerful enzymes that escape into the joint lubricant and damage joint tissue. Gold shots can, to some extent, control these harmful enzymes, it seems. This information comes from a book called *Trace Elements—How They Help and Harm Us,* by Joan Arehart-Treichel.

In his book *Overfed but Undernourished,* Dr. Curtis Wood, Jr. takes up the "fad" of wearing copper bracelets to prevent or cure arthritis. He reminds us that all statements from official sources declare unequivocally that copper bracelets or other jewelry for alleviating arthritis are "one of the oldest medical swindles." Anyone who advertises copper bracelets for sale with any mention of possible health benefits takes the risk of being investigated by the Post Office, The Federal Trade Commission and/or the Food and Drug Administration.

However, says Dr. Wood, he knows many highly intelligent people—physicians, lawyers, business executives and their wives—who wear the copper bracelets and believe they are helping. "For any cult or type of 'fad' to persist for any length of time it must have *some* merit to it," he says. Then he discusses an article published by a New York State University physician, Dr. Donald A. Gerber, who stated that "copper prevents the breakdown of protein which eventually results in the inflammatory process of arthritis."

Recent tests showed that something in the physiology of the arthritic seems to "bind" free copper so that it is not available to the body. Half of a group of arthritics suffered from this disadvantage, while only two per cent of a group of healthy people had it. Dr. Gerber said he hoped that a diet could be devised to reduce the amount of the copper-binding substances in the body, hence to prevent or treat the inflammatory process of arthritis.

Dr. Wood believes—and we agree with him—that if a substance in the body which binds copper and makes it unavailable contributes to arthritis, then perhaps putting more copper into the diet might prevent deficiency, hence prevent arthritis. It is known, says Dr. Wood, that some minerals can be absorbed through the skin. Before antibiotics were available, mercury and bismuth, two trace minerals, were rubbed into the skin as a cure for syphilis. Perhaps copper, too, can be absorbed by the skin—from a bracelet, for example.

On the other hand, Dr. Carl Pfeiffer in his fine book, *Mental and Elemental Nutrients,* says that the mechanism of whatever relief gold therapy gives is quite unknown and that the side effects such as serious skin rashes and depression of the formation of red and white blood cells can occur. If the dosages are well individualized, these side effects can be avoided. But we still do not know how or why gold injections tend to alleviate suffering from arthritis. And, of course, the patient has to return to his doctor periodically for the injections. Does the gold interfere with other trace elements which may be in excess in the joint tissues, he asks. Does gold act to alter the immune response?

He goes on to say that the typical arthritic has a copper level twice that of normal people and an iron level only one-half of that of healthy people. This seems to disprove utterly the theory that absorbing copper through the skin or taking copper supplements might be helpful. The arthritis patient has plenty of iron in joints, lymph nodes and other tissues. It's just in joints that iron is excessive. "Perhaps the excess iron in the joints may give rise to the painful inflammatory response," he says.

Speaking of lead, Dr. Pfeiffer tells the story of a man who was exposed to lead pollution only while he was cutting his way through a brick wall that had been painted with lead paint. He breathed in a great deal of lead-contaminated dust and had rheumatic symptoms in all his joints five days later. Large doses of vitamin C relieved his symptoms quickly. Dr. Pfeiffer says this is because vitamin C causes lead to be excreted. "With an adequate nutritional program, his recovery continues."

He describes another patient with "pitifully deformed hands and feet. She had not responded to steroid (hormone) or gold therapy and, in spite of a full aspirin schedule, each movement was like walking on her eyeballs." The level of copper in her blood was 238 micrograms per cent as against a normal level of 110 micrograms. Her zinc level was 78 micrograms per cent against a normal of 100. One year later, says Dr. Pfeiffer, her weight had risen from 100 to 115 and her copper is a normal 114 percent. Her zinc and iron are still low, but "her active disease process is arrested."

Another patient lives in an area where the drinking water naturally contains lots of copper, so much that the water has a metallic taste. Each summer she suffers from aching and swollen joints and frequent migraine headaches. Relatives who drink the same water also have arthritis complaints.

"Some claim that the copper bracelet, worn by the arthritic patient, will relieve joint pains," says Dr. Pfeiffer, who is a psychiatrist. "Maybe the copper bracelet is a solid clue and will be more effective against arthritis when it is made from the actual excess copper taken out of the patient's blood and tissues.

"Since copper in the serum rises because of lack of zinc and manganese in the diet and blood, we usually find these two essential elements to be low," says Dr. Pfeiffer. He points out, too, that lack of sulfur in the diet may predispose to excessively high copper. All rheumatoid patients should have zinc, manganese, niacin (vitamin B3) and vitamin C with two eggs a day, he says, since the eggs are rich in sulfur. The yolk contains more sulfur than the white, so it should always be eaten.

Other trace elements that are in very short supply in the bodies of arthritis patients are: molybdenum, chromium, tin and aluminum. From many parts of the world, according to Dr. Pfeiffer, we get reports of high iron content in drinking water resulting in many cases of rheumatoid arthritis. In laboratory analyses it appears that most of the iron is in the joints, for blood levels may be very low. In some laboratory experiments arthritis can be induced by injecting iron salts into the joints.

Yet we read that iron deficiency anemia is often a symptom of arthritics. How does this happen? Dr. Pfeiffer says that just getting too much iron in the body may result from some inability of the digestive tract to screen out iron that is not needed by the body. It is easy to tell if you have such a disorder. Taking iron supplements should soon result in the appearance of very dark-colored stools, if iron is being discarded and eliminated in the feces.

Yet people who drink a lot of iron-containing red wine or people who continually take tonics containing large amounts of medicinal iron are likely to find the iron accumulating in unexpected niches in the body like the synovial membranes, which are disordered in arthritis. "Studies have shown a disturbance in iron metabolism among arthritic patients. . . . it is possible that the synovial membranes are acting as storage depots for excess iron."

Dr. Pfeiffer believes that the weakness and fatigue which are generally supposed to be caused by iron deficiency may instead result from lack of B vitamins and/or zinc. Continuing to take tonics loaded with iron is not the best idea, if this is so. He insists on the beneficial effects of eggs in the diet of arthritics. "In clinical experience," he says, "we have found that patients with rheumatoid arthritis or hypoglycemia (low blood sugar) or mental disease need . . . two eggs (daily) and usually do not like eggs." Since the trace element sulfur is apparently essential for the health of the joints, "all patients with rheumatoid arthritis would do well to eat at least two eggs per day to provide adequate sulfur for their needs," according to Dr. Pfeiffer.

In 1968, Dr. William B. Bean of the Department of Internal Medicine at the University of Iowa said that there is some evidence that diets deficient in zinc may set the stage for rheumatoid arthritis. Chicks fed diets deficient in zinc developed bone enlargements and deformities that resemble human arthritis. And deficiency in zinc causes an increase in congenital deformities in animals.

CHAPTER 17

Herb Remedies for Arthritis?

FROM THE TIME the first human being crushed the first leaf and laid it to his sore finger or insect bite, people have been using herbs for treating illness. Of course, there wasn't much of anything else to use in those early days, except for magic spells and the songs and incantations of the medicine man or priest.

But, surprisingly enough, many of the ancient remedies for illness have stood the test of time. Experts in this field are eternally analyzing plant material, testing this or that ingredient of plants to isolate the element that may be responsible for the healing reputation of an herb. Today the most commonly prescribed heart drug is the powdered leaf of digitalis or foxglove, a stately garden plant with a beautiful flower. This leaf is a powerful heart stimulant, and also a diuretic (inducing urine).

Aspirin, used today to treat fever, inflammation, pain and arthritis, is acetylsalicylic acid whose chemical formula is chemically related to a compound called salicin. Fresh bark of the willow tree contains salicin, which probably decomposes into salicylic acid in the body. In any case, willow bark has been known for thousands of years for its pain-killing and fever-lowering ability. From the times of the early Greeks to the American Indians, willow bark has been the most widely used pain killer.

Arthritis is an ancient disease. There are many ancient remedies derived from herbs which have been used down through the ages. We went through eight or 10 herbals and found plants which have been used by somebody somewhere to allay the pain of arthritis, or rheumatism as it was traditionally called. According to the herbals, no one appears to present these herbs as "cures" for the disease. We believe that everyone should have full information in order to try anything that anyone else has found helpful. So here is a list of some herb remedies for the pain of arthritis.

An infusion of black birch bark: black snakeroot; the rheumatism weed (botanical name: *chimaphila umbellata*); boneset tea (*eupatorium perfoliatum*); leaves of the magnolia macrophylla tree; the root of pokeweed; elderberry juice; solanum dulcamara (bittersweet); wild yam (*dioscorea villosa*), which is also called pleurisy root or rheumatism root, presumably because of its action against rheumatic and other kinds of pain. It is notable that a member of the wild yam family was sought after for many years as a potential source of natural cortisone, the hormone which doctors often give for arthritis.

We would like to point out that the poke plant listed above and bittersweet, as well, are both quite poisonous and should not be used by the layman. Herb doctors apparently used these preparations in quite small amounts, watching their patients carefully to see that no one came to grief from the toxic compounds these plants contain.

Comfrey has been used to treat arthritis, garlic for rubbing the painful spots, ginseng, hawthorn, lemon, oil of myrrh liniments, myrtle (vinca), sarsaparilla, and plantain used as a poultice. Indians crushed polypody fern and rubbed the juice on the painful joints.

Burdock seed or root has been made into a decoction by

boiling two ounces of fresh root in three pints of water. Horseradish has been used. Other plants listed by the same author are alstonia bark, balm of gilead, bamboo briar, birthwort, black willow bark, blue flag, bryony, camphor, celery, chaulmoogra (an East Indian tree), cloves, coffee (yes!), black cohash, fireweed, juniper berries, kelp, *lycopodium* (club moss or ground pine), olive, paraguay tea (maté), sassafras, turpentine, white bryony (also a purgative and emetic) and buchu.

Dandelion and rosemary, carrot, celery and parsley juice or cucumber, watercress and tomato juice have been recommended. An ancient book called *Meals Medicinal* recommends many of the above remedies, plus asparagus water; seaweed extract; camomile; cider; cress and green mustard leaves, freshly grown; oil from a fir tree to rub in; powdered mace; marjoram; mulberry; mustard oil; spirits of nutmeg; rue leaves; strawberries (a source of salicylates, says the author of *Meals Medicinal*); sulfur as it occurs in radishes, cabbage, mustard and turnips; thyme (apply the bruised herb); and walnuts. The final recommendation of this physician, whose book was published in 1905, is "whale cure—body immersed in carcass of dead whale up to neck by its ammoniacal vapors." His other suggestions seem to be much more practical.

Probably the most authoritative book in this field, *American Medicinal Plants*, by Charles F. Millspaugh, lists these plants as one-time remedies for the pain of rheumatism: white baneberry, penny-royal, and *Collinsonia* or stoneroot. It is called this because its root was also used to treat kidney stone. Henbane, which Millspaugh tells us is quite poisonous. He quotes several ancient Greek herbalists who dwelt lengthily on its toxic qualities. From its name, one would assume that it is toxic to chickens. In 1905, tobacco was being used as a treatment for rheumatism. Millspaugh describes its effects and calls it "the base of the most widespread of all narcotic habits." And in the 73 years since his book was published how that habit has grown!

Today, no one prescribes tobacco as a treatment for rheumatism. It seems possible that its narcotic properties may have given this leaf its reputation as a pain killer. It dulls the senses, surely, it raises blood sugar temporarily while one is smoking it and that tends to make one feel better. Today we are far more occupied with getting tobacco addicts to stop smoking.

In one of the herbals we consulted, there is this note from an old friend of the health food movement, Dr. W. J. McCormick of Canada. Writing in the *Archives of Pediatrics* for April, 1955, Dr. McCormick stated, "I have treated a number of rheumatic fever patients with intravenous and oral doses of vitamin C from one to 10 grams daily (that's 1,000 to 10,000 milligrams). Recovery was routine in from three to four weeks. No cardiac complications. Those with incipient arthritis were given ascorbic acid (vitamin C) therapy and similar results achieved. It seems to me that articular cartilaginous lesions (disorders of the joints and cartilages) common to all rheumatic diseases are referable to nutritional deficiency of vitamin C." Could it be that the success of old-time herb doctors resulted at least partly from the vitamin C content of their freshly gathered herbs?

Maurice Mességué, an herbalist to whose home in France many rich and famous people travel to be treated for their ills, has some suggestions for herbs to use in "rheumatism" as he calls arthritis. Four slices of lemon, one pinch of lavender and one pinch of couch grass root boiled in a quart of water. Four cups of this tea should be drunk every day, he says. And he suggests alternating it with another tea made of one pinch of camomile, one pinch of lavender, two pinches of dried violets and two pinches of sage blossom—all this boiled in one quart of water.

He also believes firmly in the powers of crushed cabbage for drawing out the pain of any inflammation (could this be its vitamin C content, we wonder?). Chopped cress or chard softened in boiling water may be used as a pack on a rheumatic joint, he says. He also uses peppermint, violet leaves and black briony. Camomile, marjoram and savoury may be distilled into oil to rub on the aching spots. A hot bath in which you've put some sage and rosemary will help, he says.

Mességué says that an Englishwoman is treating arthritis with bee stings, as are scientists in Germany and the Soviet Union. It is a carefully controlled procedure, both as to the number of stings and the parts of the body involved. "It is an interesting fact that the incidence of rheumatism is remarkably low among bee-keepers and honey producers," he says. "Short of one's keeping one's own hive, it might be a good thing to gently stroke a bee from time to time."

Mességué's comments about bee stings remind us of the physician in Florida who announced some time ago that our epidemic of heart and circulatory troubles has come about because most of us are almost never bitten by mosquitoes these days. Either we don't frequent places where there are mosquitoes, or we go only to sprayed areas, so our blood never gets the benefits of the powerful anticoagulant in mosquito venom. We don't recommend that anyone set out to collect as many mosquito bites as possible, nor do we suggest getting bitten by a bee. But there seems to be considerable evidence that bee venom may protect from pain by calling out the body substance histamine. It stimulates visceral muscles, dilates capillaries and stimulates salivary, pancreatic and gastric secretions.

Histidine is being used in some research centers as a treatment for arthritis, we suppose because it decomposes into histamine in the body. Dr. Abram Hoffer, the Canadian psychiatrist who uses the B vitamins and vitamin C in treating many disorders, including our most serious mental disease, says that niacin (vitamin B3) produces a flush in some people because of its action in "calling out" histamine. This leads us to wonder if plain niacin might not be effective in alleviating arthritis. We have more to say on histidine and niacin in relation to arthritis in other chapters.

Here is a list of the herbals we consulted in writing this chapter. There are many, many more and most of them have some suggestions for allaying the pain of arthritis.

The Way to Natural Health and Beauty by Maurice Mességué, published by Macmillan in New York City; *The Compleat Herbal*, a paperback, by Ben Charles Harris, published by Larchmont Books in New York; *The Rodale Herb Book*, published by Rodale Press, Emmaus, Pa.; *American Medicinal Plants* by Charles F. Millspaugh, published in paperback by Dover, New York City; *Nature's Medicines*, by Richard Lucas, published by Parker Publishing Company, West Nyack, N.Y.; *Using Plants for Healing* by Nelson Coon, published by Hearthside Press; *Common and Uncommon Uses of Herbs for Healthful Living* by Richard Lucas, a paperback published by Arco Publishing Company, New York; *Meals Medicinal* by W. T. Fernie, M.D., published by John Wright and Co., Bristol, England (and long out of print); *Earth Medicine-Earth Foods* by Michael A. Weiner, published by Macmillan Company, New York; *Lelord Kordel's Natural Folk Remedies*, published by G. P. Putnam's Sons, New York; *Early American Herb Recipes*, by Alice Cooke Brown, published by Bonanza Books, New York; *Encyclopedia of Medicinal Herbs* by Joseph M. Kadans, N.D., Ph.D., a paperback published by Arco Publishing Company, New York; *Health Foods and Herbs* by

HERB REMEDIES FOR ARTHRITIS?

Kathleen Hunter, a paperback also published by Arco.

When using herbal remedies, keep in mind that many are quite risky. We have mentioned a few. These should be used with great care, if at all. Remember, too, that herbs are not miracle drugs. It takes a long time, usually, to achieve improvement when you are using herbs alone. The vitamins, minerals, trace minerals, enzymes or whatever it is that brings improvement must have certain cumulative effects in your body. You can't restore a good trace mineral balance overnight after years of neglecting it.

CHAPTER 18

The Value
of Yucca

To AMERICAN INDIANS in the Southwest United States, the yucca plant growing in the desert was second in importance only to water. They used all parts of it. Flower petals, seeds, seed pods, fruit, shoots, leaves and roots were eaten. "They were eaten raw, baked, boiled, made into flour, prepared and stored for future food needs in times of shortage, and as a syrup sweetener or herb tea. It has been folklore that the Indians found the yucca helpful in rheumatism as one of the many herbs handed down by generations," say Bernard A. Bellew, M.D., and Joeva Galaz Bellew in a booklet, *The Desert Yucca*. The booklet is available from Spa City Graphics, Desert Hot Springs, Calif. 92240 for one dollar.

The Bellews go on to say, in regard to arthritis, "It has long been felt that some intestinal toxicity is a common problem in cases of arthritis. For example, diverticulitis of the colon is a common finding along with constipation, or even chronic loose or watery stools. Also, arthritis has been known to follow cases of food poisoning with diarrhea or dysentery caused by pathogenic (harmful) bacteria or their toxins."

A botanical biochemist, John W. Yale, Ph.D., studying

the yucca plant, came to believe that it might be beneficial to intestinal health and, hence, to arthritis patients. The yucca steroid saponin is a harmless herb and is, in fact, not absorbed in the intestines. So Dr. Yale offered some yucca tablets to a California arthritis clinic, where it was decided to begin a one-year study of the tablets to see if they had any effect on arthritis patients.

"In brief," say the Bellews, "the yucca steroid saponin proved favorable in a sufficient per cent of cases that it justifies its use in the overall management of arthritis. Also it proved to be nontoxic as expected, since it has long represented a food and herb source of desert Indians."

The report of the results of the Bellews and Dr. Robert Bingham, Medical Administrator of the National Arthritis Medical Center and Desert Hot Springs Medical Clinic in Desert Hot Springs, California appeared in the *Journal of Applied Nutrition*, Fall, 1975.

Fifty patients with arthritis took the yucca tablets and 51 patients took a tablet which resembled the yucca tablet, so that neither patients nor doctors knew which patients were getting the yucca and which were getting a placebo or "nothing pill."

The youngest patient was 11 years old, the oldest was 92, both with bone, joint and cartilage destruction. Most of the patients were adults, many past middle age. "Since most arthritics require a wide array of medication for arthritic complaints and non-related problems," say these authors, "no attempt is made to correlate such into the results of this study. Many were taking cortisone type medication, some were taking an unknown Mexican medicine and some gold therapy in addition to analgesics (pain killers) and others." The yucca was an additional pill which they took.

More than half the patients had osteoarthritis. Less than half had rheumatoid arthritis. The disease had been present for from two months up to 42 years, with an average of 14.6

years. From two to eight tablets were taken daily, the average being four. They were taken from one to nine weeks in one group, from one to 15 months in another group. They were taken with meals, before meals or just after meals. Eleven per cent of the patients thought the yucca had improved their "gas," 12 per cent said their constipation was improved and about 75 per cent noticed no change in their elimination.

In commenting on overall beneficial effects, after the trial was over 49 per cent of the patients believed they had been helped, 28 per cent said they had felt no effect, and 23 per cent could not decide whether they had or not.

Sixty per cent said they felt less swelling, less pain and less stiffness, 39 per cent noticed no difference. Questioned as to whether they wanted to go on taking the tablets (which certainly indicates whether or not they felt improved), 47.5 per cent said yes, 27.3 per cent said no and 15.2 per cent were uncertain. The cost would have been five dollars a month for the yucca tablets. Ten per cent said they would like to take them if money was available.

The patients taking yucca were tested periodically for possible ill effects. There were no allergic reactions. There were no changes in blood condition. In some patients blood levels of cholesterol were lowered. "Since this observation was not anticipated prior to the study, follow-up cholesterol levels were not a part of this study," say the authors. "However, because medicine is still searching for a safe, effective means of lowering blood cholesterol levels, the reporters offer this chance observation, however slight."

Throughout the test period, it seemed impossible to find any systemic effects of the yucca tablets. That is, they did not appear to make any change in any important function of body organs. So it appears that yucca is not absorbed in the intestine. Then why take it? How could it possibly benefit anyone if none of it ever gets into the bloodstream?

Apparently its action is effective only in the intestine, affecting only the intestinal bacteria. These are the living organisms which inhabit our intestines, some of them friendly, some of them very unfriendly. "Therefore," say the authors, "yucca saponin would appear not to have a direct systemic effect on arthritis or collagen diseases, but rather an indirect effect, probably through enhancement of the enterocolic flora." That is, the various bacteria that live in the small intestine and the colon.

The Bellews say in their booklet, "While conceivably some patients may exhibit early relief in days, to one degree or another, it would appear that the yucca saponin has its best effect over a longer period of time. Being a saponin, and therefore a soap, the yucca saponin could be referred to as an intestinal soap or cleanser, a detergent, a wetting agent for the intestinal flora. It may well aid and abet the intestinal enzyme systems, a significant factor in health. . . .

"The results reported above, of the safety and effectiveness of yucca saponin in promoting a better intestinal flora and improvement in arthritis, surely suggest its use in the many other entercolic diseases (that is, diseases of the inside of the colon) acute, subacute and chronic. Certainly there can be no harm in investigating it and trying it on at least a trial-run group of patients. There appears to be nothing to lose but the disease. For example, many patients complain of a little burning or irritation of the rectum and anus. In one such case, (we) dispensed the yucca saponin to observe its effectiveness in this area, plus or minus. It relieved the problem almost overnight in an 87-year-old woman and the problem did not return. So it would appear that gastro-enterologists might do well to look into this area of application of the yucca saponin extract tablets."

The authors also believe it might be worthwhile to use yucca for patients who have chronic gall bladder disease or who have had their gall bladder removed and also for those who have high blood cholesterol. This could possibly replace to some extent the necessity for bile salts and cholesterol to be excreted into the intestine in gall bladder disease, or after the organ has been removed.

"This particular problem has plagued our population for many generations," say the authors.

What about taking yucca on your own for your arthritis? It appears to be completely harmless. We have taken the tablets for several months without any unpleasant side effects, for we like to try any new products before writing about them.

And just to be certain about the absolute safety of yucca, we wrote to Dr. Robert Bingham asking him if, in his opinion, it is safe to take these tablets without any medical supervision.

Dr. Bingham assured us that the yucca product is apparently not absorbed into the intestine. "It acts only in the gastrointestinal tract to reduce the colonies of harmful bacteria and parasites, according to the information we have from our manufacturing laboratories and from our clinical experience with yucca extract over the past four years.

"... While most of the good results are of the 'testimonial' type, we are conducting experiments which seem to show that there is a definite effect in arthritis, reducing pain and stiffness—probably from cutting down toxic absorption from the intestines. It also seems to help such widely related conditions as high cholesterol, headaches and migraine.

"It also works for race horses who show joint stiffness so there must be something more to it than a psychological effect.... We have probably given out 100,000 tablets and in the present dosage of six a day we have had no patients with complaints of allergies, gastrointestinal upsets or any harmful effects which we can detect."

Speaking of stress, Dr. Bingham tells the story of a young arthritic patient who came to his clinic. She was a teacher in a neighborhood where disciplinary problems made her life extraordinarily stressful. She was tired all the time. She smoked. She didn't get enough sleep or exercise. She was on a "diet" to reduce. She was taking no food supplements. A diet history showed that she was getting only a bit more than half the recommended amount of protein she should have had. She was getting too much fat at meals. She was deficient in every vitamin and mineral.

This is the program she was put on at the clinic:

1. A high protein diet with refined carbohydrates eliminated, as well as all processed and preserved foods and high fat food. She got plenty of certified raw milk, fresh fruits and vegetables, nuts and wholegrains.

2. She got vitamin supplements which gave her about four times the recommended daily allowance.

3. Her mineral deficiencies were treated with chelated minerals, especially chelated magnesium.

4. She was given yucca extract tablets which are made from the desert plant.

5. She was given an arthritis vaccine.

6. She was given female hormones by injection, later by mouth.

7. She had physical therapy of hot wax baths for hands and wrists plus hot packs and ultrasound for her knees.

8. She had therapy two or three times daily in the hot mineral waters of Desert Hot Springs.

9. She did some sunbathing and tanning.

10. She exercised, swimming and walking, gradually increasing the distance.

11. She was given a new antiprotozoal drug for three weeks.

By the end of four weeks, she was greatly improved.

Swelling of joints, stiffness and limitation of movement and pain were relieved. Dr. Bingham points out that one reason for this speedy return to health was that she came to the clinic before extensive damage had been done to her joints and before she had taken any aspirin or other drugs for her arthritis.

"On careful questioning," says Dr. Bingham, "almost every patient can date the onset of their arthritis symptoms to some single illness, injury, period of ill health or physical stress. To the nutritionally aware physician the common denominator in the onset of the disease is the period when the patient's body was depleted of proper nutritional support, lacking in the amount of food, then quantity of food and the nutritional value of food—thus lowering the patient's resistance to arthritis . . . rheumatoid and osteoarthritis don't 'just happen.' They develop only in patients who are nutritionally deficient because of poor dietary habits or recent metabolic imbalance caused by disease, injury or operation. Good nutrition prevents arthritis and provides natural resistance against the disease."

To explain the presence of an antiprotozoal drug, Dr. Bingham is following the leadership of a British physician, Dr. Wyburn-Mason, who has found a minute organism, a protozoa, in the tissues of patients with active rheumatoid arthritis. He treats it with an antiprotozoal drug which is available in England but not in the United States. He says the protozoa can live indefinitely in human tissues. Dr. Wyburn-Mason has treated a number of patients and relieved their symptoms. So Dr. Bingham also makes use of American drugs which destroy protozoal parasites, he told a recent Symposium of the International College of Applied Nutrition in California.

Of 66 patients treated with the anti-protozoal drug, symptoms become less serious gradually until, in about four months, they have disappeared and within six months blood counts are normal. Two patients who had taken the protozoal drugs were later operated on and showed no evidence of the inflammation and infection around joints which are characteristic of this disease. Dr. Bingham stresses the need for intensive nutritional support during all this treatment.

The vaccine which Dr. Bingham gives is not a new idea, he says. For many years experts in the field of rheumatology have believed that arthritis must be triggered by an infection. Various vaccines have been used in the past. At present the FDA has not approved vaccines for arthritis. Dr. Bingham states that many experts have theorized that the pain and inflammation of arthritis, like many other chronic infections, "represent the result of long continued sensitization to bacteria and antigen absorption from foci of infection, particularly in the nose, throat and gastrointestinal tract." Only about one-third of the patients given vaccines have shown permanent benefit. Dr. Bingham thinks those who have not responded or those who must take "booster shots" must have some hidden infection somewhere which has not been located or treated, probably in the digestive or intestinal tract.

Dr. Bingham summarizes his position thusly:

"Arthritis can be successfully treated, arrested and occasionally cured utilizing available modes of therapy, if every available mode of therapy is included to its maximum benefit. A change to a quiet, peaceful environment and a warm desert climate is often beneficial. The use of natural hot deep mineral pools to improve circulation and to permit comfortable joint motion and exercise is valuable. Conventional methods of physical therapy, hot paraffin baths for the wrists and hands, hot packs and ultrasound for the joints and active gymnasium exercises as well as walking and swimming are prescribed. The medical history is important, particularly the ingestion of brackish water, possibly containing pathogenic (toxic) protozoa.... Newer treatment methods include the use of Yucca as a food supplement, arthritis vaccines to improve the patient's immunity to infections, and anti-protozoal drugs.... The use of megavitamin therapy and minerals, particularly vitamin A, D, calcium are essential to rebuilding of the bone and joint structures in arthritis patients. Further progress in the treatment of all forms of arthritis and prevention of most arthritic diseases are based on *applied nutrition*, exercise, careful medical management and treatment of the patient as a 'whole person.'"

With regard to yucca, we don't recommend giving up a good diet and diet supplements in order to take nothing but this desert plant. Arthritics need all the help they can get from diet and diet supplements, as well as other helpful therapies. We don't recommend giving up any therapy your doctor is using, if you have found it helpful. Dr. Bingham's experiments were carried out on patients who were using other therapy as well, including physical therapy like hot mineral baths, swimming, special exercises and so on.

But there seems to be no reason not to add yucca to your other aids in trying to combat arthritis. Southwest Indians, using it over thousands of years, would have been well aware of any potential dangers, it seems certain. Perhaps you are one of the many who can and will benefit from yucca. There seems to be no reason not to try it. It is available in easy-to-take tablets.

CHAPTER 19

Alfalfa and Arthritis

A MORE OR LESS official book, *Nature's Healing Arts*, published by the National Geographic and written by Lonnelle Aikman, describes some of the uses of plants for treating arthritis, recipes that have endured through many generations of mountaineers. These quotes come from natives of the Appalachian Mountain chain in Eastern U.S.A.

"For arthritis, make a tea from either the seeds or leaves of alfalfa.... Place a spiderweb across a wound.... For diarrhea, drink a little blackberry juice...."

On another visit to a mountaineer's cabin, author Aikman describes the herbs grown and used every day by the Rasnick family.

"Invited into his house," says Ms. Aikman, "I had a sip of homemade cough syrup much less fiery than the poke remedy he makes for arthritis. Besides its base of boiled horehound leaves, stems and blossoms, it contained wild cherry bark and berries, anise seeds, red clover, sugar and a touch of whiskey—and it tasted fine.

"I also met Mr. Rasnick's paralyzed wife, Joyce, whom he looks after tenderly. 'I make a tea for her out of the blossoms, stems and leaves of the alfalfa you saw blooming,' he said. 'That's for her arthritis. She has a doctor who gives her diuretics for a weak heart. There's also a medicine for the same thing made from wild grapevine root.'"

The idea that alfalfa products are therapy for arthritis—at least for some people—runs through folk medicine. We have picked it out often from collected articles on arthritis. We have heard it from friends, relatives and others who have used it to advantage. The encounter with the Rasnicks reported above shakes our faith in folk healing, we must admit. If, indeed, Mr. Rasnick was taking such good care of his family by feeding them all manner of folk remedies, why was his wife paralyzed, why did she have heart trouble and why did she have arthritis?

The mountain people are poor folks, generally. Chances are they have not much in the way of a nourishing diet, especially high protein foods, which are expensive. It's certain that they have no access to any food supplements which might contribute a lot in the way of vitamins and minerals. In winter the amount of vitamin C available must be very little indeed, for fruits, berries and fresh vegetables are probably unobtainable.

Under these circumstances, it's good that folk medicine is still practiced among the mountain people. Herb teas, while not good sources of vitamin C, undoubtedly contain many minerals and trace minerals that are of inestimable value.

Arthritis has been linked to too much sugar in the diet, a circumstance that almost guarantees diabetes in susceptible individuals. If the two diseases are closely related then it appears that alfalfa tea may be valuable for its manganese content.

Recently we saw a clipping from a newspaper in Pennsylvania, which included a column by Dr. H. Curtis Wood, Jr. The subject was "Alfalfa and Arthritis." Dr.

ALFALFA AND ARTHRITIS

Wood, a physician, is the author of the book, *Overfed but Undernourished.*

Dr. Wood says that many people find remedies for their arthritis which the Medical Establishment scoffs at. Why not, he asks. "Marked improvement and even cures have been widely reported by arthritis sufferers who are convinced of the effectiveness of their particular remedy, even if their doctors are skeptical and tend to attribute the improvement to something else.

"If one believes that washing in the river Jordan cured a man of leprosy, why might not faith in alfalfa cure arthritis?" he reasons. "Psychosomatic factors can be very powerful."

He goes on to describe the case of a cousin and long-time friend of his, Mrs. A. B., "whose honesty and integrity is beyond question." He believes her story, he says, even if it seems like a miracle.

In 1969 she developed numbness in her left hand and arm and persistent neck pain. Not until 1971 did she seek help from a New York physician. His X-ray studies showed severe osteoarthritis of the cervical vertebrae. By 1977 she had much more pain, although she wore an orthopedic collar, did many exercises prescribed for arthritics and used formula pain pills.

Visiting friends, she asked about a big bottle of pills on the dining table. Her host told her that he had cured a shoulder pain and a back pain which he had had for 28 years by using alfalfa tablets. He took two 10-grain alfalfa tablets at each meal and was completely free from this long-standing pain in both back and shoulder.

Mrs. A. B. bought some alfalfa pills and began to take them. Within five days, she reported to Dr. Wood, she began to feel better and in a week she was almost free from the pain and numbness. After six months she told him she was still free from pain and did not need the collar or the pain pills.

As almost always happens in cases like this, her doctor noted her great improvement and said, "Well, that alfalfa must contain something your system needs."

Dr. Wood had the alfalfa analyzed and found that it contains 18.9 per cent protein, plus the following vitamins: A, B complex, C, D, E, K and U, along with these minerals: aluminum, magnesium, phosphorus, chlorine, sulfur, silicon, sodium and potassium. It is also a source of several digestive enzymes, he says, and chlorophyll, which may play some role in the healing process.

Is alfalfa then a cure for anybody's arthritis? "We humans are all different," says Dr. Wood, "and our needs are different, so what helps one person with a certain disease may not help another. Genetic factors are involved, and it is interesting to note that Mrs. A. B. has an aunt and a brother, both of whom had symptoms similar to hers; both have been helped by taking alfalfa tablets.

Dr. Wood goes on to ask that any reader of his article who has arthritic symptoms and tries alfalfa with or without success should write and tell him about their experiences. "We might start a little clinical research program."

Dr. Wood suggests that you get the alfalfa tablets at the health food store, take two after each meal, "but give the program a try of at least two months before evaluating it. Don't expect to duplicate the miracle, one-week results reported by Mrs. A. B. Alfalfa tablets are cheap and harmless, so what is there to lose?"

We agree. Only we would suggest waiting longer than two months to evaluate results. And we would earnestly urge any reader who tried the alfalfa to combine it with a diet in which sugar and every food that contains it have been eliminated, where high protein meals are the rule, along with ample food supplements containing plenty of the B vitamins, vitamin A and minerals and trace minerals. Manganese and zinc, along with vitamin C have been mentioned many times in relation to the health of collagen, which is what is disordered in any arthritic disease.

You may write to Dr. Wood in care of The Chestnut Hill Local, 8434 Germantown Ave., Philadelphia, Pa. 19118.

CHAPTER 20

Arthritics
May Have a
Zinc Deficiency

IN 1968, Dr. William B. Bean of the Department of Internal Medicine at the University of Iowa said that there is some evidence that diets deficient in zinc may set the stage for rheumatoid arthritis. Chicks fed diets deficient in zinc develop bone enlargements and deformities that resemble human arthritis. And deficiency in zinc causes an increase in congenital deformities in animals.

A physician from Seattle, Washington has been treating arthritic patients with a daily zinc supplement given with each of the day's three meals. He reports that results have been encouraging.

The Lancet for September 11, 1976 contains an article by Peter A. Sinkin, M.D., of Seattle, describing a trial of zinc supplements for 24 of his patients with "refractory" rheumatoid arthritis. This means arthritis which did not respond to any other method of treatment. It was a double-blind experiment.

That is, the volunteers were divided into two groups. One group was given their regular medication plus zinc supplements for 12 weeks. The others got their regular medication plus a tablet which contained nothing. Not until the end of the trial when all observations on joint swelling, morning stiffness, walking time had been made and the patients themselves described how they felt, was the code broken so that patients and doctor alike knew which had received the zinc supplement.

The doctor examined all patients at the beginning of the trial, recording scores for swelling of joints, tenderness in each joint, along with scores for the length of time morning stiffness persisted, and grip strength, as well as ability to walk 50 feet in less than 30 seconds. Patients reported any symptoms they had of such things as discomfort, nausea, vomiting, change in appetite or bowel habits and so forth. X-rays of all hands were taken at the beginning of the test, again at 24 weeks.

Says Dr. Sinkin, "patients taking zinc sulfate fared better in all clinical parameters than did patients receiving placebo (the nothing pill)." In every area investigated—swelling, pain, stiffness, walking time, the ones getting the mineral improved while those who did not take the zinc showed little or no improvement. The only test in which the zinc did not seem to bring much improvement was the grip strength. An early improvement in the test group was not sustained, says Dr. Sinkin.

After the original test, all the volunteers in both groups were given zinc supplements and all reported improvement. There were few side effects. Headache, rash, change in appetite, abdominal pain or discomfort and diarrhea were all reported oftener in the group *not* getting the zinc supplement than in the group which got it. All side effects were mild, however.

The zinc sulfate was taken after meals to prevent any difficulties with nausea. Dr. Sinkin suggests that it would be preferable to take a zinc supplement which would be better absorbed and would be taken without any digestive irritation. "From our experience," he says, "and that of others, virtually all patients can tolerate oral zinc sulfate for three to six months. Possible toxic effects of prolonged use must still be carefully sought." He believes that much additional work must be done to confirm his observations and to determine what part zinc plays in the health of joints.

All the various conditions that are grouped under the head of arthritis diseases are also called "collagen" diseases, since it is the connective tissue which is disordered or inadequate in these conditions.

Zinc seems to be extremely important in regard to collagen—its formation and its good health. In a book on trace minerals, Volume 1 of a series called *Trace Elements in Human Health and Disease*, deals with the trace minerals zinc and copper.

In a chapter on collagen, the authors, Felix Fernandez-Madrid, Ananda S. Prasad and Donald Oberleas, discuss the effects of zinc deficiency on the creation of this connective tissue called collagen. They describe experiments which show that the effect of zinc deficiency on the manufacture of collagen is a generalized effect on the manufacture of protein and on the workings of nucleic acid, rather than a direct effect on the manufacture of collagen.

For example, deficiency in zinc produced (in laboratory rats) a great decrease in the amount of three amino acids or forms of protein in the skin of the animal. These three amino acids (glycine, proline and lysine) are especially important ingredients of collagen. So lack of zinc, resulting in a lack of these three kinds of protein, could be very important, indeed, to the health of the skin, as well as other tissues.

This suggests, does it not, that anybody with any kind of skin condition might notice improvement by simply increasing the zinc in his or her diet. It also suggests that the almost universal complaint of skin ailments these days—especially among teenagers—may have a lot to do with lack of zinc in their diets.

"The daily intake of zinc may furnish or be slightly below the human requirement," says Walter Mertz, U.S. Department of Agriculture, Nutrition Institute. "Recent research already has identified population groups that are at risk of marginal or deficient intake. Although the available data are still limited, they alert us to the possibility that marginal zinc deficiency may not be uncommon in the United States. This recognition led to the fortification by the Food and Nutrition Board subcommittee. It is already implemented by most of the infant food manufacturers."

It is well known that wounds do not heal as quickly as they should in living things which are deficient in zinc. Giving zinc improves this situation. Zinc accumulates at the site of an injury, which seems to demonstrate that the body sends it there to help in healing, as white blood corpuscles are sent immediately to a wounded area to help in healing.

It is well known, too, that children who are deficient in zinc do not grow as they should, which seems to indicate that they do not have enough of this trace mineral to help them make the protein necessary for all the collagen in bones, cartilage and other connective tissues. "In general," say the three authors, "studies of a variety of connective tissues in the zinc-deficient state have shown conclusively a significant reduction in the total collagen in the zinc deficient state."

People deficient in zinc also show abnormalities in the way the body uses those important substances DNA and RNA, which are the elements in cells which regulate heredity. As each cell divides, it takes with it part of the original RNA and DNA, so that the next cell will be normal. These substances are also made of protein. If zinc is essential in making protein, then it seems likely that the creation and operation of RNA and DNA (also called nucleic acids) would suffer.

It seems, indeed, from several reports, that zinc participates in the manufacture of nucleic acids—RNA and DNA. In animals made deficient in zinc the body manufacture of DNA was impaired. DNA is necessary for cells to divide. Cells must divide in order to create collagen. So the breakdown of this entire process seems to be implicated in reduction of collagen which develops in animals deficient in zinc.

There is every reason to believe that the same thing happens in human beings. Lack of zinc causes disordered collagen health and inefficient repair. Now think, for a moment, of the many parts of the body which are likely to suffer from such a circumstance. Most of all, think of the millions of Americans imprisoned in a "collagen disease" of one kind or another—rheumatoid arthritis, osteoarthritis, gout, lupus erythematosus, rheumatic heart disease in children, and so on, through the whole dismal catalog of ills.

At present many millions of Americans suffer from some form of collagen disease. According to the Arthritis Foundation, about 97 per cent of all Americans over the age of 60 have collagen diseases of greater or less severity. In other words, these diseases are almost universal among older folks.

Doesn't it seem quite possible that one reason, at least, for this epidemic is the fact that practically all the zinc is removed from that group of foods which make up about half of most American diets—the refined carbohydrates—and is never replaced! Since these are the foods in which zinc is quite plentiful, it seems likely, does it not, that people who have eaten real wholegrain breads and cereals and have eliminated white sugar from their diets early in life are much less likely to suffer from the arthritic diseases than those who continue, throughout life, to eat white bread, exclusively, plus desserts, processed, sugary cereals, soft drinks, candy and so on, to the exclusion of most foods which contain any zinc at all.

In 1973, testifying before a Senate Select Committee, Dr. Walter Mertz, Chairman of Human Nutrition Institute of the U.S. Department of Agriculture, said, "We have not yet learned to understand the optimum requirement for all essential trace nutrients. Therefore, if we fabricate our own foods, we must accept that our knowledge is incomplete and therefore it is entirely possible that our fabricated foods are inferior in quality to that of the more wholesome products . . . we certainly have an example in zinc nutrition. In the past 5 to 10 years evidence has accumulated that the zinc nutrition status of a proportion of our older population is not optimal as shown by very good effects of increasing their zinc intake."

He went on to describe one of the commonest symptoms of zinc deficiency—lack of or impairment of a sense of taste. One survey showed that 8 to 10 per cent of supposedly normal children from middle and high income families were markedly deficient in zinc, as shown by the fact that their taste sensation was deficient, and they lacked appetite. Lack of appetite is very common among older folks. And often it is accompanied by the complaint, "I just don't seem to be able to taste anything any more."

No one, so far as we know, has correlated these complaints with arthritic disease. That is, we cannot prove that arthritics are deficient in zinc, since this lack of appetite and sense of taste is one of the chief symptoms of zinc deficiency. But why wait until someone performs all the laboratory work necessary to make such a deduction?

Why not be sure to get enough zinc now, every day, in order to prevent arthritic diseases, if they threaten you, or perhaps alleviate them if you already have one or another of these painful conditions?

Foods which contain the most zinc are seafoods—fish and shellfish. How often do you eat them? After that come the wholegrains and cereals, as well as all seed foods and nuts. But only real wholegrains—remember that. Zinc has been removed from any and all processed cereals, as well as white flour. Use only wholegrain cereals—the kind you get at your health food store. There, too, you can get the best in the way of seeds of all kinds, and nuts—all rich in zinc.

Other good sources of zinc are meat, especially liver, eggs, brewers yeast, peas, carrots, brown rice and milk. Do you include all these regularly in family meals? If not, you are likely to produce zinc shortages in members of the family, especially the older ones. And remember that every time you use white sugar or any food containing it, you are diluting the trace mineral quality of your diet, including zinc, for this food is devoid of any minerals at all. So don't waste any space on your shopping list for refined carbohydrate foods of any kind.

Officially adults need about 15 milligrams of zinc daily. If you are not sure you are getting enough of it at meals, your health food store has zinc supplements.

If you suffer from arthritis, there is no reason to delay in taking a zinc supplement. There is no need to take the sulfate form which Dr. Sinkin gave to his patients. Your health food store has zinc supplements which are readily absorbed. These come in various potencies, marked on the label. An especially valuable kind is the "chelated" product, meaning that the mineral has been associated with amino acids which "chelate" it into a form which is much more readily absorbed by the body.

Dr. Sinkin's patients were taking large amounts of zinc

three times daily. Much more zinc would undoubtedly be absorbed from a chelated product than from the zinc sulfate tablet which Dr. Sinkin gave. So there seems to be no need to take as much as he was giving patients in his experiment. Eat lots of those foods which contain plenty of zinc and avoid those from which it has been removed. And take a zinc supplement. It is a perfectly natural substance which cannot harm you.

CHAPTER 21

A Distinguished Nutrition Expert Speaks on Arthritis

"INJURIES, INFECTIONS, allergic reactions and psychological stresses may all play a part in the cause of arthritic disease, but the most probable underlying cause—poor nutritional environment for the cells and tissues involved—has, as usual, been neglected," says Dr. Roger J. Williams of the University of Texas in his fine book, *Nutrition Against Disease.* It is published in paperback by Bantam Books, New York.

He quotes a comment from a supposed "expert" at *Consumer Reports,* who dismissed the whole subject of vitamin pills, saying, "Healthy people who eat balanced diets don't need them." Dr. Williams points out that this may be true in the case of perfectly healthy people who eat perfectly balanced diets. He personally does not know any perfectly healthy people. He mentions deformed and retarded babies, hardening of the arteries (which is almost universal in our society), heart disease (which may appear at an early age), obesity and overweight (which afflict possibly half of our population), dental disorders (which are universal), stiff and disabled joints, mental disease, addiction to drugs, alcohol and tobacco. He asks, as we have asked many times, "where are the perfectly healthy people? Who are they?"

His motto, he says, is always "If in doubt, try nutrition first." He thinks this is probably very true in the case of the arthritic group of diseases.

The synovial fluid which bathes all joints and movable parts of our bodies consists of water, minerals and a mucoprotein made by our bodies. To manufacture this protein our bodies must have available all the ingredients that are needed. Any cook can understand that, if you are making raised bread, you must have flour and fluid of some kind plus yeast and a number of other ingredients. If you lack even one of these—the yeast, let's say—the resulting product is a sorry counterfeit of what you had in mind. And no matter if you provide the finest flour and other ingredients in exact proportions, without the yeast you will get a soggy mess of bread hardly worth trying to salvage.

It's the same with nutrition. "If any mineral, amino acid (protein) or vitamin is in deficient supply, or if the cells are poisoned by bacterial toxins or allergens, this can partially incapacitate the cells and can lead to poor lubrication, with every movement accompanied by friction and pain," says Dr. Williams.

He then reviews the spectacular results that have been achieved by some physicians in the past who have used nutritional therapy for the arthritic diseases. Dr. William Kaufman (discussed in another chapter) used niacinamide (a form of the B vitamin niacin) in very large doses, tailored to the needs of each individual patient. His patients reported amazing improvement, in some cases complete amelioration of symptoms. It did not happen overnight. And enough of the vitamin had to be taken—very, very large doses.

Pantothenic acid, a B vitamin discovered and named by

Dr. Williams, has been used by British physicians to treat arthritis, as we report in another chapter. They discovered that the level of pantothenic acid in the blood of arthritics is only about half that in the blood of healthy people. Those people who had even less pantothenic acid than that were even more severely crippled and in some cases bedridden. Experiments with this B vitamin have continued to the present.

Many patients with arthritis suffer from anemia, says Dr. Williams. Another B vitamin, folic acid, brought relief from pain to 20 cases of rheumatoid arthritis, although it did not change the basic condition, so it must be only a partial answer. Folic acid prevents one kind of very serious anemia. Riboflavin (vitamin B2) has been found to be lower than normal in the blood of more than half of a group of arthritics. This deficiency may be "a nutritional weak link" in the nutritional chain which produces good health. If any link is weak, the production of the lubricating fluid is disordered, says Dr. Williams.

Other researchers found that arthritics have less of vitamin A in their blood than non-arthritics. "It is not at all impossible that its lack may cause arthritis conditions," says Dr. Williams.

He mentions the work of Dr. John Ellis, the Texas physician who has used vitamin B6 (pyridoxine) for his arthritic patients. Dr. Ellis reports some success in relieving pain, stiffness and unlocking finger joints. The vitamin also helps to prevent numbness in arms and legs, night cramps, pain in shoulders, hips and knees. He prescribes 50 milligrams a day of pyridoxine. Dr. Ellis does not claim that vitamin B6 "cures" arthritis. Dr. Williams believes that this vitamin may be still another link in the nutritional chain which keeps most of us safe from this painful disorder. All the links are important.

Some years ago, Dr. Williams tested minerals in nine

healthy young men eating "their customary diet." He analyzed their urine, blood and saliva for these minerals: sodium, potassium, calcium, magnesium and phosphorus. The average levels of sodium varied by 6 per cent. Calcium and phosphorus levels varied by 30 per cent and the magnesium level in one man's body was more than 200 per cent higher than in another. It has been discovered, says Dr. Williams, that the calcium "needs" of normal young men vary about five-fold. (Some may need five times more than others). A study of bone densities (indicating the strength and health of bones) reveals enormous differences. This certainly indicates, Dr. Williams believes, that proper mineral balances must always be considered on an individual basis. Your needs for any given mineral may be far higher than the average person's.

Cholesterol deposits and hardening of arteries often accompany arthritic diseases. Part of the reason for this could be lack of the mineral magnesium. Part of the reason, we believe, could also be too much sugar in diets and too little exercise to help wear off some of the bad effects of the sugar.

Uric acid is supposedly the body product which produces gout. We are supposed to produce too much uric acid as a result of "high living"—too much of the wrong kind of food. But, says Dr. Williams, he has tested uric acid levels in co-workers and has found that very high levels of uric acid may be present without any gout symptoms. "The mere presence of high uric acid in the blood is not enough to cause gout; its salts must be precipitated in and around the joints, and this does not always happen in individuals who have a high content of uric acid in the blood."

And, according to Dr. Williams, there is evidence that vitamin C is probably most effective in treating and preventing back and neck pain. He thinks its usefulness here arises from its essential nature for maintaining the structure of the intervertebral discs. Almost everybody these days suffers from disc trouble. A doctor in Texas uses vitamin C in gram-a-day doses for all his patients with back problems and reports success.

Why? Dr. Williams refers back to one of his favorite themes: biological individuality. Each of us has his own characteristic nutritional needs for various nutrients. They remain with us through life. Those with back and neck pain throughout life may simply be suffering from lack of enough vitamin C since their needs may be higher than the average person's.

"I certainly would not want to give the impression that the management of these diseases is simple," says Dr. Williams. "But I do reaffirm the dictum that nutrition should be tried first. On the basis of reports presently available, the items that certainly need to be considered are niacin (vitamin B3), pantothenic acid, riboflavin (vitamin B2), vitamin A, vitamin B6 (pyridoxine), vitamin C, magnesium, calcium, phosphate (phosphorus) and other minerals. The objective is to feed adequately the cells that are involved in producing synovial fluid and in keeping bones, joints and muscles in healthy condition."

Dr. Williams' wise recommendations on arthritis make up one chapter in his fine book, wherein this distinguished nutrition researcher recommends what he calls "supernutrition"—a condition, he says, which no living being on the earth has yet experienced—including human beings.

It's a condition in which nutritional need is met with enough and more than enough of every nutrient. Now for the first time in all of our history on this planet we can aspire to such a glorious state of health, for we know what essential foods to eat. We have, in this country, enough of them, and we have a vast store of knowledge of which nutrients can be added to a good diet to improve health even more.

Dr. Williams calls this concept "supernutrition" because it signifies a kind of health insurance which will take care of any excessive needs for nutrients which you may have due to inheritance, diet or way of life.

CHAPTER 22

Is Arthritis
Related to
What You Eat?

"... WHAT WE EAT today is 'food' almost completely devitalized, with its important and necessary ingredients largely battered, heated, frozen, or pulverized out of it, and with a very few of them—barely understood and not at all coordinated—then needled back in along with dozens of other substances which ought to play no role in human feeding at all. And if the Mad Scientists do manage to include in their needles a substance that is actually related to food, they gleefully assure us that the food from which they have taken all but a drop of life is now 'enriched,'" report Gene Marine and Judith van Allen in *Food Pollution—the Violation of Our Inner Ecology* (Holt, Rinehart and Winston, New York, 1972).

If you agree with this rather pessimistic appraisal of our food supply, as we do, then you can readily see how such debilitating diseases as arthritis entrap thousands of Americans each year. If you are eating an unvaried diet to begin with, and much of the food you are eating is depleted of essential nutrients, then you can more or less expect to eventually succumb to disorders such as arthritis. Such a non-nutritious diet is bound to be deficient in essential vitamins, minerals, proteins, etc.

Medical World News for February 14, 1964, reports on a study conducted by the National Institutes of Health on two groups of Indians in the West: one living in warm desert country, one living in the cold regions of Montana. Although there seems to be some evidence that arthritics improve in warm climates, it was found that the Indians living in the hot desert region had more arthritic complaints than those who lived in Montana.

Speculating on reasons for this, the researchers considered such things as infections and heredity. Neither seemed to explain the situation. They found that the arthritic disorders were present mostly in desert Indians of a certain age group. Looking back in history, they uncovered the fact that during the time these people were children they had experienced "a deficient nutritional status in infancy" because of drought and famine.

Even among the Montana Indians, those who grew up during a period of food shortage in their part of the country showed more cases of the disease than those who were older or younger. There seems to be no doubt that lack of proper nutrition in infancy and childhood is involved.

We know that most American children today do not lack food. There is an abundance of food. But with practically nothing to guide them to nutritious foods, and with every resource of advertising used to persuade them to eat non-nutritious, empty-calorie foods, it is not surprising to find that many rather young people these days, especially young women, are developing rheumatic diseases.

A Washington physician reported on cases of inflammation of tissues of the shoulder and other joints occurring in people whose thyroid glands were not functioning properly. When this was cleared up, the disorder disappeared. Five British physicians reported in a January, 1964 *British Medical Journal* that they had discovered deficiency in folic acid (a B vitamin) and vitamin B12 in a group of arthritic patients. They proceeded to take careful histories of exactly what these patients ate every day and of the reserve store of vitamins in their blood.

They found that the arthritic patients consistently got less vitamin C at their meals than a similar group who did not have arthritis. They also tended to take smaller amounts of iron, protein and total calories. At all age levels the reasons for this were simply that they did not eat enough foods containing these essential nutrients.

They found, too, that the average content of folic acid in the arthritic patients' diets was about one-fifth of that in the average British diet. Once again, these sick people just didn't eat foods that contain this B vitamin. Wouldn't you say that such a finding almost certainly indicates some relation between diet deficiency and arthritis?

Surely it is time that some of the research money poured into government grants and independent foundations be used to study the past diets of the many millions who suffer from this disease to determine if there is some kind of pattern which recurs in most of them. Some interesting things might emerge. Perhaps there is dislike of fresh foods. Or a tradition in the family that desserts must be rich and frequent. Perhaps there is an over-emphasis on starchy and sweet foods with not enough high protein and vitamin-rich foods eaten every day. Perhaps the diet contains too many "junk" foods and the embalmed foods referred to in the opening paragraph.

The healthy person doesn't succumb to diet disorders. The careful person doesn't take a chance on succumbing, because of past indiscretions in diet and way of life. Even though his past diet habits have been entirely adequate, he bulwarks his present health by being even more cautious than perhaps he needs to be. In regard to vitamins and minerals, the wise person takes no chances. It is better to err on the safe side.

CHAPTER 23

A Startling Theory on Arthritis

ONE OF THE most startling, not to say horrendous, developments on causes of arthritis comes from a Rutgers University horticulturist who says, in a book on the nightshade family of plants, that these vegetables are the cause of arthritis.

It's not that they are polluted with pesticides which cause the arthritis. It's not the way they are grown. It's not that one may have an individual allergy to one or another of these foods. It's just that all plants of this family of plants are naturally poisonous and contain alkaloids that bring on the aches and pains of arthritis.

Now—hold on to your hats—the following plants are members of the nightshade family: potatoes, tomatoes, peppers, eggplant and tobacco. Dr. N. F. Childers who, with G. M. Russo, wrote the book, *The Nightshades and Health*, holds a doctorate in fruit production. His research and publications are respected throughout the world, according to a recent news item in the *Chicago Sun Times*. Another of his books, *Modern Fruit Production*, is a standard reference teaching textbook in advanced level horticultural courses.

Such a statement as this coming from a man of Childers' stature could be expected to cause a stir, says the *Sun Times*. Some people in related fields of the academic community have rejected the theory saying that Childers' evidence is too incoherent, nonsensical and "flamboyantly unscientific" to be taken seriously.

Another equally qualified expert of the University of Maryland, Dr. Arthur H. Thompson, believes that Childers' evidence is "remarkable." He met Childers on a plane trip, got to talking about the alkaloids in plants of the nightshade family, and, being an arthritic, immediately eliminated all such vegetables from his meals. Within several months his 20-year case of arthritis of the lower spine was completely cured, he says.

Scientists have known of the alkaloids in the nightshade family of plants for many years. *Toxicants Occurring Naturally in Foods,* published by the National Academy of Sciences, tells us that several people have indeed died from eating potatoes. This is because of the presence of the alkaloid solanine in certain kinds and conditions of potatoes. It is concentrated in the skin and becomes hazardous only when green-colored skins are eaten *raw* or sprouts are eaten *raw*.

"All existing and newly developed varieties of potatoes are now monitored for alkaloid content," says this classic standard reference work. It goes on to say, "Past experience of man has contributed much more to our knowledge of margins of safety of natural foods than has animal experimentation.... A wide variety of common foods contain known goitrogenic (goiter causing) substances or antithyroid activity due to unknown components. Here the margin of safety, assuming a normal well-balanced diet on a chronic basis, is undoubtedly less than 10 (very low)." The same is true of other poisonous substances in plants.

We do not know if Dr. Childers, in his book on the nightshades, goes into the origin of these foods for human consumption. They come from South America. Whole nations and communities of people—whole areas of that vast continent—lived almost exclusively on potatoes, tomatoes, peppers and perhaps some corn. Some of the mountain people ate almost nothing but potatoes, as, indeed, the Irish did for many years after potatoes were introduced into that country as cheap, easily raised food for poor people.

Some South American Indians in the high mountains have been living almost exclusively on potatoes for more than 4,000 years, because that is the only food which will grow in that climate and altitude. Practically all of the thousand or so varieties of potatoes which are known today were cultivated and developed by the Indians in Peru centuries before the Spanish conquerors arrived.

As we know, South and Central America were also the birthplace of peppers. They, too, were cultivated and developed with such skill that many varieties existed thousands of years ago. To this day, they represent a large part of the diet of these southern people. They are rich in vitamin C—an excellent source, in fact.

What Italian housewife could cook without tomatoes? Although they originated in South America, they are the hallmark of Italian cookery. When potatoes and tomatoes were introduced into Europe the feeling against them was so strong that governments had to put on promotional campaigns to persuade people to eat them, for they were associated in the public mind with the poisonous nightshade family.

But, if just these three vegetables are the cause of arthritis, it seems evident that the Indians of South America could never have prospered as they did, living almost exclusively on just these plants, without any "well-balanced diet" to dilute the possible effects of any alkaloids. And certainly it seems fairly reasonable to assume that people crippled with arthritis from babyhood could hardly have performed the astonishing physical feats of these early Indians—building roads by hand through thousands of miles of wilderness; carrying messages by running over the mountains at unbelievable speeds with matchless endurance; scraping a living out of stony mountain soil with primitive tools.

How could such an active and vigorous people be universal victims of a disease that cripples and deforms, that brings anguished pain with the slightest movement?

Meanwhile, perhaps Dr. Childers has hit on something phenomenal. So, if you have arthritis, there is nothing to prevent you from trying a diet which excludes potatoes, tomatoes, peppers and eggplant. Most long-time arthritis sufferers have tried just about every diet—why not this one? It's possible, of course, that millions of modern individuals are peculiarly sensitive to the alkaloids in these foods and these may be the people who get arthritis.

If you customarily use lots of tomatoes and peppers, and decide to go on a diet which eliminates them, be sure to supply in some other food the vitamin C and the fiber which is quite abundant in these two foods. If you decide to eliminate potatoes, allow yourself some good, wholly natural source of the fine carbohydrate and protein they contain. Don't substitute sweets or refined starches for potatoes. Such a diet would prove very unwise.

The remaining notorious member of the nightshade family is tobacco. Many arthritis sufferers smoke, and we know that smoking depletes our store of vitamin C, which benefits our connecting tissues. Some people with arthritis chew tobacco and/or dip snuff, although we have no proof that the ingestion of tobacco—or other members of the nightshade family—causes arthritis. But stop using tobacco anyway!

CHAPTER 24

The Miseries of Gout

IT WAS IN 1776 that a German physician identified the body substance responsible for gout—uric acid. Later a British physician connected this substance with the disease by discovering it in the tophi. Tophi are deposits of sodium urate in the skin, near a joint. Many gout victims have them. Healthy people don't. For thousands of years in history, gout has plagued human beings, especially men, and, especially famous, talented achievers like Benjamin Franklin, Alexander the Great, Chamberlain, Lloyd George, Louis XIV, William Pitt and many more.

It is estimated that about one million Americans have gout. It is a metabolic disease, affecting the entire body but mostly announcing its presence by attacks of excruciating pain which occur suddenly and may not occur again for weeks or months. Joints of the foot are usually the most painful—the great toe is the most common site of the pain. No one knows what incident causes the first attack, or why later attacks may or may not occur.

The disease is caused by the body's mishandling of the waste product uric acid. Too much may be manufactured in the body, or too little may be excreted in urine. So it collects in tissues and circulates in blood. The purines in food are the chief source of uric acid from outside the body. The other source is the purine from the patient's own tissues breaking down, as tissues do. Trying to get rid of the urates, the blood deposits them in various spots, including the kidneys.

Other animals do not suffer from gout, since they have an enzyme which is missing in human beings, uricase, which handles the uric acid successfully. Only human beings, the ape family and, for some unknown reason, the Dalmatian dog, do not have this enzyme in their bodies. The disease appears to "run in" human families. It is most common during and after middle age. It seems certain that overeating and overdrinking are conducive to further attacks of gout after it is once established. As Dr. Darrell C. Crain says in *Arthritis Handbook*, "the gouty patient develops symptoms because his body has a basic chemical defect and cannot cope with certain foods."

Injuries to joints are one cause of attacks of acute gout. Overeating of certain foods rich in purines is another cause. Drinking excessively is another cause. Acute attacks may follow the week after an operation, even a minor one. Some medicinal drugs may also precipitate attacks. *And stress.*

"In a group of university professors given physical and psychological tests, those who had high levels of uric acid in the blood often seemed to rate higher in traits such as drive, leadership qualities and achievement," report Dr. Randolph Lee Clark and Dr. Russell W. Cumley in *The Book of Health, Third Edition.* "In another series, corporation executives had higher mean levels of uric acid in the blood than did the craftsmen. Further studies may show whether uric acid has any effect upon the reasoning centers of the brain which might explain these statistical observations."

It is recommended that sufferers from gout who wish to

keep entirely free of the disease should not eat kidneys, brain, liver, fish roes or sardines, and should not drink beer, wines or spirits, reports *The Stein and Day International Medical Encyclopedia.*

"Spinach, strawberries and rhubarb are also forbidden," the encyclopedia continues.

"Until a few years ago the only known remedy (for gout) was a drug called colchicine. Even the Egyptians, who suffered from gout along with other ancient peoples, knew about this drug," says *About Gout*, a free pamphlet from The Arthritis Foundation, 3400 Peachtree Rd., N.E., Atlanta, Ga. 30326.

"But colchicine, while it alleviates acute attacks, can produce unpleasant side effects. It is extremely powerful, and the amount needed to control an attack of gout is about the same as the amount that will cause abdominal cramps and diarrhea.... Among the newer drugs used in controlling attacks of gout are phenylbutazone, oxyphebutazone, indomethacin and probenecid ... Allopurinol prevents the over-production of uric acid which can trigger an attack of gout. It is extremely effective and its side effects are minor." (The phenylbutazone family of drugs is noted for causing extremely serious, possibly fatal blood diseases.)

In most cases the first sign of gout is the sudden appearance of pain in one or several joints, we are told by Dr. George E. Paley and Herbert C. Rosenthal in *Medigraph Manual.* These become swollen, red, shiny and tender to touch. As the attack subsides, the skin usually peels.

"During the attack, temperature may be high and there is weakness and headache," the manual reports. "Gout may also begin with the sudden appearance of kidney stones. Crystalline deposits (tophi) may be found in the skin—particularly in the ear lobes.... In the early stages of the disease the joints recover from an acute attack without permanent injury. Months or years elapse between attacks, during which time the patient is quite comfortable. However, as the disease progresses, these intervals become shorter—and chronic, gouty arthritis, resembling rheumatoid arthritis, is likely to develop."

The most serious complication of gout is a slow, progressive kidney involvement which can lead to uremia and death, the manual continues. Younger patients with gout frequently develop high blood pressure and generalized hardening of the arteries. A gout patient can become virtually crippled from the deformation, stiffening, and impaired motion of the involved joints.

At a recent meeting of medical researchers in London, a professor from the University of Glasgow said that physicians should investigate the possibility of vitamin C deficiency in patients who complain of gout. If the gouty joints show tiny hemorrhages, it's quite possible that there is nothing wrong with the patient but too little vitamin C. We know that stress destroys vitamin C rapidly, as do smoking and many other things in our environment. Could it be that gout patients have need for far larger amounts of vitamin C than the rest of us and that their attacks, after different kinds of stress (overeating or overdrinking, injuries or operations) are simply indications that more vitamin C must be provided? It's certainly worth trying.

Adelle Davis, in her book *Let's Get Well,* presents many other arguments for vitamin treatment of gout. She says that the B vitamin pantothenic acid is required to change uric acid into harmless substances which can be excreted. Experiments in which volunteers were subjected to stress showed that they developed large amounts of uric acid, which was released into their blood. If they had been given massive doses of pantothenic acid for six weeks before the experiment, the uric acid content was decreased. She suggests that whole families may have much higher requirements for this B vitamin, which would explain gouty attacks in members of the family subjected to stress. The severe stress of fasting has produced gout in some obese people, she tells us, because of high levels of uric acid.

Lack of vitamin E may also play a part. People deficient in vitamin E may have excessive amounts of uric acid. The fats in cell walls tend to be destroyed or oxidized when not enough vitamin E is there to protect them. Adelle Davis reminds us that, in ancient times, the rich and the powerful ate lots of meat. There was no refrigeration, so, of course, the fats in the meat were mostly rancid, as were butter and lard. Rancid fats destroy vitamin E wholesale. So possibly eating rancid fats resulting in vitamin E deficiency was the cause of gout in earlier days. Today we know that vitamin E is lacking in our meals because of the milling of cereals and flours. So perhaps this is the reason for an increase in incidence of gout.

Another reason for accumulation of uric acid in some individuals, according to Miss Davis, is that normally much of the uric acid produced by the body is excreted into the intestine and used by the healthful bacteria that live there. If these have been destroyed by oral antibiotics, chances are that uric acid will accumulate. This suggests that good sources of the helpful bacteria (*lactobacillus acidophilus*) should be available at all times. Yogurt and buttermilk are good sources, and many preparations of these bacteria are available at health food stores. It's true, too, that a high fiber diet is conducive to the growth of the friendly intestinal bacteria. So getting lots of fiber in meals and snacks is advisable. Fresh fruits and vegetables in goodly quantity are essential. All breads and cereals should be real wholegrain. Unprocessed bran is the best source of fiber.

Adelle Davis refused to plan diets which were low in

purines, for gout patients, for, she said, people who came to her for diet planning had demonstrated that wheat germ, yeast, liver and other foods usually totally forbidden on the low-purine diet, had been especially helpful in preventing gout attacks. If the doctor has absolutely forbidden purine-rich foods, she says, then at least vitamin E and the B vitamins should be taken in large amounts.

Miss Davis also suggests that the gout patient pay special attention to keeping his diet more than nutritionally adequate and taking vitamin C and the B vitamin, pantothenic acid, with him at all times, to take "with protein food" every two or three hours during times when he is under special stress.

In its leaflet—*Gout, A Handbook for Patients*—the Arthritis Foundation states, concerning diet, that no diet can eliminate all the substances from which the body manufactures uric acid, so dieting is "an imperfect method at best." Then, a diet low in purine is so different from the patient's usual diet that he may not want to follow it for long periods of time. And, finally, restricting the purine in meals is of little or no value in preventing the sudden, acute, painful attacks of gout.

Some further notes on gout: lead poisoning can induce it, as shown by the widespread occurrence of gout in moonshiners who drink whiskey distilled in lead containers. Calcium and many other nutrients help to protect against lead poison. In a 1967 study, highly significant correlations were found with alcoholic consumption and gout—especially consumption of beer. Smoking was also much more common in gouty people. Because of the heavy excretion of uric acid, the gout victim is also subject to kidney stones and other kidney damage, due to deposits of urate. It's interesting in this connection to remember the many physicians who give large doses of vitamin C to prevent kidney stones. Even 20 years ago, a Canadian physician was using massive doses of vitamin C to prevent kidney and bladder stones.

The involvement of kidneys in excreting uric acid suggests that drinking large quantities of fluids (water, fruit juice, milk) can help to prevent kidney damage from urates. Many of us, especially as we grow older, tend to forget the importance of drinking plenty of fluids to prevent kidney and bladder infections, as well as stones and other disorders of these organs of elimination. With the gout patient, it seems that drinking large amounts of fluid every day is especially important.

What about sugar? In his provocative book, *Sweet and Dangerous,* Dr. John Yudkin, the eminent British researcher, tells about studying gout and rheumatism patients in two or three clinics.

"As we half expected," Dr. Yudkin says, "the patients with rheumatoid arthritis were eating the same amounts of sugar as control subjects. But the patients with gout were taking appreciably more sugar than the control subjects; the median values were 102 grams of sugar a day for the gouty patients and 54 grams for the control subjects."

And then there is the story of Dr. Ludwig W. Blau, Ph.D., who, more than 20 years ago, discovered that eating cherries (any kind) dispelled the attack of acute gout from which he was suffering. He told his doctor, who put some gout patients on cherries—not many, just a handful—every day.

Later Dr. Blau wrote up the results in *Texas Reports on Biology and Medicine*, Fall, 1950. He reported on 12 cases of gout which responded favorably to cherries. The uric acid of the gout victims dropped to normal and no further attacks of gout appeared in these 12 patients, even though they were on unrestricted diets. They ate about one-half pound of cherries every day. They were canned cherries, sour cherries, black, sweet, Royal Anne or Bing. One of the patients drank cherry juice with equally good results.

No one in the medical establishment paid any attention to Dr. Blau's discovery, so far as we can determine. But eight years later, *Food Field Reporter,* in its November 10, 1958 issue, told of gout patients getting relief from drinking canned cherry juice. This was the result of a commercial firm in Wisconsin experimenting with their own produce among a number of local residents suffering from gout.

"To date," said *Food Field Reporter*, "there is no definite scientific data on just how the juice aids in relieving pain caused by diseases where improper balance of calcium is evident. However it is believed that it may be the pigment in the cherries that brings relief." Cherries contain several pigments, also a considerable amount of pectin which some arthritic sufferers have found to be helpful in alleviating the pain of arthritis. Cherries also contain various acids (citric, oxalic, succinic and lactic acid).

The Arthritis Foundation reports that no one, to their knowledge, is doing any experiments with cherries or cherry juice in relation to gout. That is what one would expect. Cherries, like other food, cannot be patented as a remedy for any disorder. Drugs can be. A vast amount of money can be made by a drug company which produces a drug that millions of gout sufferers will require. Nobody in the business of raising cherries has any money for conducting tests, nor is there any indication that medical science would pay the least bit of attention to the results, no matter how promising they might be.

There is no reason why you cannot try eating cherries or drinking cherry juice if you suffer from gout. There is no indication that cherries will interfere with any treatment your doctor is giving you. They are good food, after all.

"The mere presence of high uric acid in the blood is not enough to cause gout; its salts must be precipitated in and around the joints, and this does not always happen in individuals who have a high content of uric acid in the blood, "reports Dr. Roger J. Williams in *Nutrition Against Disease*.

"One of the time-honored measures to be taken in the case of gout is to avoid consuming food that contains substantial amounts of nucleic acids (sweetbreads for example), because nucleic acids give rise to uric acid in the body. Nucleic acids and uric acid, like cholesterol, are produced in the body (endogenously), however, and their avoidance in food may not effectively prevent uric acid piling up in the blood or its salts from being precipitated to settle in the joints," Dr. Williams says.

He adds that the same measures that may be used to prevent arthritis may also be used to prevent gout. Gout is closely related to arthritis, and in some cases arthritic deposits are suggestive of gout. There is nothing which prevents people from having both gout and arthritis at the same time, he says.

CHAPTER 25

Arthritics May Not Be Able to Tolerate Gluten

THERE'S A DOCTOR in Australia who believes that rheumatoid arthritis may have something to do with inability to deal with the cereal protein called gluten. Dr. Raymond Shatin of the Alfred Hospital in Melbourne created a stir at a meeting of specialists in rheumatic diseases a number of years ago when he announced this theory and backed it up with maps of areas of the planet where gluten-high cereals are eaten. The areas correspond, he says, to areas where rheumatoid arthritis is most prevalent. And the disease is not very common in localities where rice and corn (both low in gluten) are the basic cereals.

Furthermore, he said, anthropologists tell us that very ancient animal and human bones they have dug up show definite evidence of the related disease, osteoarthritis. But human bones and joints affected with rheumatoid arthritis have not been found in any "digs" dated before 2750 B.C. This was long after human beings had begun to raise their own cereals. So, presumably, the cause of the rheumatoid bones and joints might be associated with the new diet in which cereals like wheat, barley, rye, oats and buckwheat play a large part.

These are cereals in which there is plenty of protein gluten. Corn contains almost no gluten. Ancient South American Indians ate corn exclusively, since wheat, rye and other European cereals were unknown to them. The bones of these ancient South Americans show no evidence of rheumatic arthritis, says Dr. Shatin.

On the other hand, bones of long-dead Egyptians dug up from ancient tombs show evidence of rheumatoid arthritis. The Egyptians, way back then, ate lots of wheat and did not grow or eat corn. So they were getting plenty of gluten in their meals, whereas the South Americans were not.

There is no suggestion from Dr. Shatin that wheat, rye, barley, oats and buckwheat are harmful in any way to the average person. But a number of people inherit the inability to deal with gluten. That is, they simply cannot absorb it, for they lack the enzyme that is necessary for this. So it causes trouble for them, chiefly in the area of the small intestine.

Celiac disease is one manifestation of this enzyme lack. Some investigators believe that multiple sclerosis is another disease whose origins may have something to do with inability to digest gluten.

Dr. Shatin has asked the question, "Isn't it possible that those who develop rheumatoid arthritis are victims of the inherited defect? Mightn't they be able to avoid the disease by just eliminating from their diets those cereals rich in gluten?"

He gathered 30 arthritic patients to his hospital and put them on a diet from which all gluten-containing foods were eliminated. Twenty of the patients obtained relief from symptoms. Some of them for as long as 18 months. Dr. Shatin asked for more research, encouraged other scientists and physicians to conduct similar experiments.

Several researchers at Yale University took up the challenge and conducted tests. They were brief and seemed to show that there was no abnormality in the small intestine, hence no inability to process gluten. The very small group of people tested did not, during the five days of the test, notice any improvement in their arthritic condition when they were placed on diets containing no gluten.

This may or may not prove anything. Very few patients were involved in the test. It went on for only five days. In any case, there is no reason why people suffering from this agonizingly painful disease should not test for themselves what their own reaction to gluten is. There is no need to make elaborate preparations. Just eliminate those cereal foods in which gluten is most abundant, for several weeks or longer, and see what happens.

These are the cereals that must be avoided: wheat, rye, millet, barley, oats and buckwheat. These are the foods you can substitute for them: cornmeal and corn flour, rice, rice flour, soy flour, potato flour, lima bean flour, cornstarch.

The easiest plan is just to eliminate all cereals and breads for as long as you want to test the theory. There are plenty of foods to replace them: potatoes, any vegetables, any legumes, nuts, seeds, peanuts and so on. But if you want to go to some trouble, make your cereals and breads out of the cereals and flours listed above. Any all-rice breakfast cereal is permissible. You can make hot breads from cornmeal, soy flour, rice flour or lima bean flour. It takes a bit of extra effort.

If you suffer from rheumatoid arthritis, you may find that such a diet relieves your symptoms. You may find that it does not. You have not wasted your time; you have participated in a worthwhile experiment and proved something worth knowing. If you should be interested in going on a gluten-free diet because of arthritis or any of the other conditions in which intolerance to gluten is involved, there's a dandy book available which gives many recipes for gluten-free foods to make at home. It's called *Good Food, Gluten Free* by Hilda Cherry Hills. It's published by Keats Publishing Company, New Canaan, Connecticut. It's a paperback for $3.50.

CHAPTER 26

Do Weather
and Stress
Influence Arthritis?

IN 1962, a distinguished specialist in rheumatic disease, Dr. Joseph Lee Hollander of the University of Pennsylvania, went to a great deal of trouble to discover, if he could, how much weather conditions influence the course of rheumatoid arthritis.

He constructed a large room in which he could produce any weather condition he wished. Into it he put some volunteers suffering from rheumatoid arthritis. These people lived there for several weeks, going about their usual activities. It was a kind of vacation for they spent all their time in the test room without going to work. They read, sewed, played games, slept, ate and visited with one another.

Meanwhile, back at the controls which had been constructed, Dr. Hollander experimented with many weather changes of which the volunteers had no warning. He tried to make the room cooler, warmer or more humid. He changed the air pressure in the room, from time to time, without mentioning these changes to the volunteers. None of these changes seemed to make a bit of difference in the symptoms of the people being tested.

For a while, according to a New York paper which reported the story, Dr. Hollander doubted the claims of arthritics that they can prophesy the weather by how their joints feel. Then he remembered that patients seem to suffer more when a storm is coming. So he used his elaborate equipment to produce something like the beginning of a storm. He kept the temperature constant but increased the humidity and dropped the barometric pressure.

Almost at once, 29 out of the 40 patients reported that their arthritic symptoms were worse. The increasing pain and stiffness were not imaginary. They were real and could be proven by well known tests for stiffness, tenderness and strength of grip. Varying just the humidity or just the barometric pressure brought no changes in symptoms. But changing both to simulate the way things feel when a storm is coming made all the difference.

Dr. Hollander believed that his experiments demonstrated why arthritic patients feel better in Arizona or some other locality where there is little rain and low humidity. Arthritic patients in places like these do not get the sudden changes in two or three aspects of weather which are frequent occurrences in parts of the country like the Northeast, where such changes happen often, summer and winter.

So it is possible for an arthritis patient to predict a coming storm with some comment like, "My knees are beginning to ache again. We're in for some bad weather."

The *British Medical Journal*, commenting on experiments of this kind, said, in 1964, "Most people who have studied the effects of artificially mild climatic conditions have found that change of weather is sometimes associated with onset of pain. An equable climate is therefore perhaps of some value although it does not seem to play a very important part in the genesis of the disease itself. Most people feel more at ease in a warm, moderately dry climate without extremes of temperature, and the same is true of rheumatic sufferers on average."

The Arthritis Foundation, discussing the matter of weather, says, "A more favorable climate does not cure the disease. Many patients are more comfortable, however, in a warmer area where there are fewer weather changes. A permanent move or winter vacation should be discussed freely with the patient's physician and if there is any hardship involved it may not be worthwhile. It is also true that some patients react favorably to a colder climate."

The Foundation also says, about spas and warm mineral springs, "The spas offer a place of relaxation with controlled exercise and rest. The warm pools provide buoyancy and heat and in them the arthritic can move more freely. These are indeed important attributes. There is no good evidence that the mineral content of the water taken either internally or externally has any beneficial effect."

And what about stress, emotional factors, resentment, personal disasters? Do these play any part in the onset of arthritis or its continuing course?

The Arthritis Foundation says, "Emotional upsets, tensions and shocks apparently play some part in rheumatoid arthritis. Symptoms sometimes begin after a disturbing event. In patients who already have the disease, it may seem to get worse during periods of upset and better when such stresses are relieved. This is not to say that emotional or psychological factors *cause* rheumatoid arthritis, but only that they may contribute to the problem in some way."

Adelle Davis in her lively and stimulating book, *Let's Get Well*, says "Arthritis remained a mystery until it was shown that remarkable results were obtained when cortisone was given. Obviously, if the body were producing all the cortisone it needed, further cortisone could bring no improvement. Such results indicated that persons with arthritis were in the exhaustion stage of the stress reactions . . . and that their pituitary and/or adrenal glands could no longer function normally. Since this knowledge became available, the arthritic individuals with whom I have worked have often improved remarkably after following a diet designed to stimulate natural cortisone production and to meet the increased nutritional needs of stress."

She then emphasizes the need for greatly increased amounts of protein taken in small frequent meals. The B vitamin pantothenic acid can scarcely be overemphasized, she says. "Prolonged stress increases the nutritional requirements so much that deficiencies of pantothenic acid and/or vitamins B2 or C can be produced and cause the adrenals (glands which help us to handle stress) to become severely damaged, hence several weeks may be necessary for repair before improvement can be expected."

She goes on to report that animals under stress sometimes need 70 times the normal requirement for vitamin C to protect the health of the adrenal glands. Calcium is withdrawn from bones when the individual is under stress, so plenty of calcium is needed. She recommends two grams (2,000 milligrams) of calcium daily from dairy products and from supplements.

In addition, Adelle Davis used to insist on diets loaded with nutrients. Liver every day or desiccated liver tablets if liver could not be eaten. Wheat germ for breakfast cereal. Green leafy vegetables in abundance. Enormous doses of the B vitamins and vitamin C taken frequently during the day, plus 100 unit capsules of vitamin E and twice daily a capsule of 25,000 units of vitamin A and 2,500 units of vitamin D. She insisted that no refined foods at all be eaten (sugar and white flour products), no hydrogenated fats, no coffee or alcohol.

She says that the nutrients which must be emphasized are the same regardless of whether the diagnosis was rheumatoid or osteoarthritis, bursitis, spondylitis or other classifications of the arthritic disease.

Furthermore, Adelle Davis believed that arthritis can be a psychosomatic illness. That is, resentment, anxiety and long-buried conflicts, hostility and deprivations can produce actual joint swelling and pain. She believed that the person with arthritis may have had more to be angry or hurt about than the rest of us. She tells, in this book, almost unbelievable stories of testing people who came to her for a diet program that would help their aching joints.

One woman came creeping in, obviously in great pain, to tell Miss Davis she had suffered from arthritis for many years and had spent thousands of dollars on doctors' bills. Adelle Davis placed a large pillow in one corner of the room and asked her to kick it "to improve her circulation." The woman kicked it with great vigor and then attacked it with her fists, screaming threats and cursing. For 10 minutes she kept this up, then returned to her chair and found that she could not only sit down without pain but could also get up easily and walk easily. She came back after three weeks of practicing this same kind of "exercise" at home and Davis hardly recognized her. Almost no pain or stiffness remained.

It occurs to us that releasing some pent-up emotions may be the reason so many people find gardening helpful to health. It's very vigorous work. You work out any hidden resentments or anger pulling weeds, turning over soil, trundling heavy wheelbarrows, lugging stones, sawing wood and so on.

A study reported in *The New York Times* in 1963 told of three separate sets of twins, one of which, in each set, had arthritis while the other did not. One set consisted of 26-

year-old nurses, one of whom left nursing to get married and have a baby. She lived with a hostile mother-in-law who was paranoid. The situation was so difficult that she left her child with the mother-in-law and went back to nursing. Very soon she developed rheumatoid arthritis in her fingers and arms. Her twin stayed healthy.

Another set of twins were 51-year-old unmarried women, one of whom was "trapped" at home with a near-psychotic stepfather and a sick mother. She always felt under tension. She had severe arthritis. Her twin sister was well. The third set are college-educated women, one of whom has an unsuccessful husband and no children. She is crippled with arthritis. The other twin is not.

The two physicians who presented this study said these cases confirmed their continuing study of 100 arthritis patients: that there are characteristic personality patterns and stressful experiences in patients that precede the onset of the illness.

The same year the Southern California Chapter of the Arthritis and Rheumatism Foundation presented the findings of the national medical director of the Foundation which dwelt on the almost total lack of arthritic disease among prison inmates. "These individuals who let out their anger and aggressive feelings so violently that they wound up behind bars, had practically no rheumatoid arthritis."

There seems to be little doubt that stress—especially prolonged stress without any let up—can bring on arthritic pains. It also seems quite clear that rest, relaxation, vacations, getting away from the stress in whatever way is best for you can relieve arthritic pains and, to some extent, repair the damage. The lesson to be learned seems to be to avoid prolonged stress whenever you can. Some stress is unavoidable. But get away from it whenever you can, as soon as you can. And, if it appears the stress will continue, bulwark yourself with all the nutritional helps you can manage. The adrenal glands wear out rapidly under continual stress.

A reader of one of the nutritional magazines that we edit, troubled by arthritic pains in her knees, told us she noted almost immediate improvement when she went on a 3-week vacation in Vermont. She walked several miles a day in Vermont with no pain. She wondered if the arthritis might be caused by pollution and water fluoridation in the big eastern city in which she lived.

In other chapters we discuss the possibility that lead pollution may cause arthritis; also that exercise is of great help to many arthritics. What about water fluoridation, which is found in many city water supplies?

Dr. H. A. Cook was talking of fluorosis in the October 9, 1971 issue of *The Lancet*, a British medical journal. "A high intake of fluoride is known to cause severe skeletal fluorosis," said he, "but the actual fluoride intake required to produce fluorosis is unknown. I have shown that tea-drinking in Britain causes a high fluoride intake in both children and adults, maximum intakes in children surveyed reaching nearly 6 milligrams daily in unfluoridated areas and nearly 7 milligrams daily in fluoridated areas. It is possible that fluoride intake from tea may be sufficient to cause fluorosis, and I report here a case which gives some evidence of this."

He then described the case of a 55-year-old woman who had been crippled with arthritis for 25 years. Twelve years earlier she had moved to an area with more fluoride in the drinking water, since she had been told by her doctor that fluoride is good for teeth and bones. The water here contained 0.67 parts per million (ppm) of fluoride or just about half the 1.5 ppm recommended in our country for municipal drinking water. The arthritic woman drank from 3 to 4 pints of tea daily, or roughly 6 to 8 cups.

A urine test showed that she was excreting 1.5 to 2 ppm

of fluoride, which, according to authorities quoted by Dr. Cook, indicates that fluoride is being retained—that is, bones and teeth are taking it up from the water and incorporating it into bones and teeth.

The arthritic woman stopped drinking tea. Within three months, she told Dr. Cook, her arthritic pain had diminished to the point where she was almost able to do without the drugs she had been taking for 25 years. She was able to move about so painlessly that she took a job involving lots of walking. Within six months she was virtually free from pain and doing without drugs entirely.

One year after she stopped drinking tea, there was no further improvement, but there was also no deterioration. She could do without drugs entirely except in emergencies. "Possibly," said Dr. Cook, "some cases of pain diagnosed as rheumatism or arthritis may be due to subclinical fluorosis which is not radiologically demonstrated." He means it cannot be seen on X-ray pictures.

Tea—plain, supermarket tea—is relatively high in fluoride. The amount you get in any cup of tea depends on how strong the tea is and how long you allow it to steep. There are probably also differences in the amount of fluoride in different kinds of teas, although we have never seen any figures on this. If your drinking water is fluoridated, this, of course, adds fluoride to the cup of tea. If you forget about the teakettle and allow it to boil and boil away before making the tea, this concentrates the fluoride, so there is more of it in such a cup of tea.

It is interesting to note that the reader who told us her story about freedom from beginning arthritis pains when she went to Vermont lives in a city where the water is fluoridated.

The Lancet article does not involve herb teas. So far as we know, there is no excessive amount of fluoride in any herb tea, assuming you are using unfluoridated water. But we should not forget that we are exposed to fluoride in many kinds of environmental pollution, aside from drinking water. And it's the total intake that causes the damage, if any. In any case, it is another form of stress that we can do without. Perhaps some of us can get along healthfully on more fluoride than others. There is great variation, of course, in individual reactions to any poison. And fluoride, in large enough amounts, is a poison.

CHAPTER 27

For Foot Health, Go Barefoot!

AN ORTHOPEDIC SURGEON, Paul W. Brand, states firmly that the person who goes without shoes will have much healthier feet than the one in shoes, in spite of occasional wounds from stones, thorns or broken glass.

Some of the foot disorders that the barefoot walker avoids are: corns, hammer toes, bunions, hallux valgus (a deformity of the great toe), metatarsalgia (pain and tenderness in the metatarsal region), ingrown toenails and athlete's foot. And maybe even arthritis!

"There is a sense of aliveness and joy walking barefoot that I never get in shoes," says Dr. Brand, who has studied foot problems for almost 30 years in India, England and Ethiopia. When he was working in an orthopedic clinic in India, he noticed that the only patients with ankle fractures were people who wore shoes. He constructed a device to test the ability to detect a slight tilt of the ankle which might produce a fracture. His barefoot patients could feel the tilt immediately. Those who wore shoes took longer to react. "If you're wearing shoes, you can't feel a rock underfoot as well, so it may be too late to react to the tilt," says Dr. Brand. Platform or heavy-soled shoes compound this problem by minimizing the wearer's control.

ARTHRITIS

Indian and Pakistani hockey teams played barefoot for many years, to allow for quicker reflexes and greater speed. They won a number of gold medals, according to *Medical World News* for November 15, 1976. But they had to put on shoes when they met opposing teams whose studs and cleats tore their bare feet to ribbons.

Many pediatricians prescribe stiff shoes for toddlers to help them from the crawling to the walking stage. Dr. Brand points out that the children would do much better and develop much better muscle control if they were allowed to go barefoot all the time they are growing up. "It's bad enough that adults deform their feet, but it's criminal for them to do it to children," he says.

Of course, the city dweller must choose the places he can walk barefoot with safety. Even in his own home or on his own lawn, he may encounter furniture, stones or other obstacles that may injure his feet. A smooth, sandy beach is surely the best place of all to walk barefoot. Meadows, fields, forest and lawns were all traversed by many thousands of barefooted ancestors of ours who either had no shoes or preferred to go barefoot. There is evidence that their feet were healthier than ours, for it's our shoes that produce the painful deformities we mentioned at the beginning of this chapter. There's never a bunion, a hammer toe, a corn or an ingrown toenail on the foot that has always been barefoot.

The one exception to Dr. Brand's rule is the diabetic or the leper who has lost sensation in the feet, hence is unable to prevent injuries or even know that he has suffered one. A past president of the American Diabetes Association reminds us that even a tiny cut on the diabetic foot can lead to infection, as can tight shoes, causing corns or blisters. Dr. Brand believes that the wrong shoes can cause almost as many injuries and ulcers in diabetics as would foot injuries.

FOR FOOT HEALTH, GO BAREFOOT!

Drs. Malcolm I. V. Jayson and Allan St. J. Dixon, both M.D.s, in their book, *Understanding Arthritis and Rheumatism* (a Dell paperback), tell us that many of the complications that develop in these sufferers have their beginning in the wrong shoes. "Shoes cause more foot problems than anything else," they say, "and faulty shoes are especially to blame. If we didn't wear shoes there would probably be about 90 per cent fewer foot troubles than are suffered today.... Ideally the child should grow up in an always equable climate and do nothing but run around in bare feet on a grass lawn all day. He would presumably grow up without any foot deformities at all," they say.

Painful feet are almost universal among us prisoners of a technological urban society. Arthritis of any part of the feet is one of the most painful and crippling of all ailments. Many different kinds of foot pain have been diagnosed. In nine out of 10 people with arthritis, the joints of the feet are involved. The joints may swell, the fatty cushion that pads the bottom of the foot may move away from the weight-bearing area so that eventually only thin skin protects the damaged joints from the hard ground. Any part of the foot may become deformed by arthritis. Even a succession of expensive, individually fitted shoes can bring little comfort to the arthritic, for changes in the size and shape of the foot may soon render any pair of shoes uncomfortable.

The older we grow the more likely we are to suffer from arthritic feet. The skin on our feet becomes thin. The ligaments inside the foot become stiff and the whole foot relatively rigid. Nails tend to thicken and become hard to cut. All earlier deformities tend to worsen. The arthritic who has trouble bending as well as poor eyesight cannot take care of his or her feet properly.

Surely one of the best ways to avoid many of these foot problems in later life is to kick off your shoes and scurry around barefoot as often and for as long a time as possible every single day. The second best thing is to ignore fashion and wear shoes that are divinely comfortable on all occasions. You should never allow a bunion, a corn, an ingrown toenail, a foot infection, for all these can and should be prevented by just choosing shoes which make you feel as if you were walking barefoot.

CHAPTER 28

What About Aspirin?

FOR HIS PATIENTS with fever and pain, Hippocrates, the Greek physician regarded as the Father of Medicine, suggested that they chew on the bark of a willow tree. Hippocrates may not have known it, but the bark contained salicin, a chemical cousin of aspirin.

The remedy worked and for thousands of years primitive people have been chewing on willow-tree bark and other barks in order to relieve pain. In the 1800s, European chemists managed to segregate the salicin from the bark for a more logical way of ingesting the substance. Later, chemists discovered two other drugs, similar to salicin—acetylsalicylic acid and salicylic acid—which were said to be stronger than salicin. In 1899, the Bayer Company began manufacturing acetylsalicylic under the trademark of Aspirin.

Today, in the United States, physicians pass out some 14 million recommendations for aspirin to their patients each year. Thus, aspirin has become the second most widely used drug. Alcohol is apparently in the No. 1 position.

If you are a victim of one of the many types of arthritis, aspirin may be one of the few ways in which you can get relief. Even so there are risks, and it will be up to you and your physician to decide which is the lesser of two evils.

In several chapters in this book we have reported that aspirin destroys vitamin C. In 1971, two California researchers—Dr. Mervyn A. Sahud and Dr. Richard J. Cohen—writing in *The Lancet*, reported that arthritic patients who took high doses of aspirin had reduced concentrations of vitamin C in their blood plasma and blood platelets. Vitamin C tablets brought the levels to within normal ranges, even when the patients were taking large doses of aspirin. Large doses were considered to be 12 or more aspirin tablets daily. This research involved 34 patients with rheumatoid arthritis.

In a recent book, *Drug-Induced Nutritional Deficiencies*, Dr. Daphne Roe reports that, in 1964, a researcher studied six patients with rheumatoid arthritis who also had the anemia caused by folic acid deficiency. The doctors then studied 46 more arthritis patients who also had deficiency in folic acid, the B vitamin. The researchers theorized that the over-growth of cells in the joints of rheumatic patients may give them an increased demand for folic acid. But Dr. Roe points out that all but three of these arthritics were taking drug combinations which include aspirin. And aspirin is known to deplete the body of folic acid.

One hazard of elderly people is the fact that they are the chief users of prescription drugs. A list of long-term maintenance drugs used by people over 65 includes drugs for arthritis, drugs to prevent blood clots and convulsion, heart drugs, blood pressure drugs, drugs to treat diabetes, water pills or diuretics, hormones and drugs to treat tuberculosis. "As previously indicated," says Dr. Roe, "many drugs in these categories are known to be capable of inducing vitamin or mineral deficiencies."

Folic acid blood levels are known to be low in a high percentage of patients with rheumatic arthritis, says Dr. Roe. In 1971, a researcher found that 71 per cent of 51 arthritic patients had low levels of folic acid. All of them were taking aspirin—we presume in large doses which is usual with arthritics. Arthritic patients who were not taking aspirin did not show low levels of folic acid.

"Three gastroenterologists told a Senate Subcommittee that antacid aspirin products—Alka-Seltzer in particular—can aggravate some stomach disorders whose symptoms the antacid remedy is supposed to relieve," reported *The New York Times*, June 7, 1973.

The witnesses stressed that consumers should be warned that aspirin and patent medicines containing aspirin may pose acute dangers to persons suffering from stomach ulcers and gastric bleeding. The specialists also took issue with the FDA, which at the time proposed changes in the content, advertising and labeling of some antacid preparations.

The testimony was given to the monopoly subcommittee of the Senate's Select Committee on Small Business.

Added Dr. Stuart H. Danovitch, chief of gastroenterology at the Washington Hospital Center, Washington, D.C., "Alka-Seltzer, as well as other preparations containing sodium bicarbonate, represents a potential burden of sodium to patients who are on a salt-restricted diet."

Heavy aspirin users may find themselves with some bigger headaches than the ones they're trying to cure: gastric ulcers, bleeding ulcers, ulcerative colitis and other intestinal problems, reported the *New York Post*, October 16, 1974. "That's the consensus of some of the world's top specialists on stomach and intestinal ailments attending the fifth World Congress of Gastroenterology (in Mexico City)."

Dr. Morton I. Grossman of the University of California at Los Angeles told the meeting that one-third of those suffering from gastric ulcers were "chronic, heavy aspirin users." He said that some victims took huge quantities of aspirin to control arthritis, but that the majority were just chronic aspirin users. "They take it for headaches and often they can't tell you why."

Dr. Atanas Maleev, deputy minister of public health and director of the Academy of Medicine in Bulgaria, said: "We have observed that 50 per cent of the bleeding ulcers, ulcerative colitis and serious lesions in the intestines seem to be directly related to patients who abuse the use of aspirin."

Dr. Humberto Romero Tocuyo of Venezuela said that the worst aspect of aspirin was that it and medications containing acetylsalicylic acid are advertised profusely and are also consumed in great quantities by the public.

Science News, September 29, 1973, stated that "Two years ago aspirin was found to inhibit prostaglandins, local hormone-like regulators in various tissues. Since prostaglandins induce fever, aspirin may relieve fever by inhibiting prostaglandins. Since prostaglandins help produce inflammation, aspirin may counter rheumatoid arthritis by inhibiting prostaglandins.

"Now," the publication added, "aspirin has been found to inhibit lymphocytes—white blood cells that constitute immunological defenses in the body." These findings were reported in the September 1, 1973 issue of *The Lancet* by P. I. Terasaki of the University of California at Los Angeles and A. A. Hirata of Abbott Laboratories.

"Aspirin's therapeutic value against rheumatoid arthritis might be partially explained by aspirin's ability to inhibit lymphocytes. White blood cells as well as prostaglandins are involved in rheumatoid arthritis," *Science News* said.

Writing in *Hypothyroidism: the Unsuspected Illness*, Dr. Broda O. Barnes and Lawrence Galton state that, "It has been said that just one-fifth of an ounce of iron stands between us and suffocation. For iron goes into the making of hemoglobin, and anemia can result when a deficiency of iron leads to a deficiency of hemoglobin."

WHAT ABOUT ASPIRIN?

Iron deficiency can stem from chronic loss of blood. In women, the deficiency may result from excess menstrual flow; in men, from the slow bleeding of a peptic ulcer; in both sexes, from hemorrhoids or piles, Dr. Barnes and Galton said.

Other possible causes, according to Dr. Barnes and Galton: large doses of aspirin or aspirin-related compounds, hiatus hernia, tumors of stomach or intestine which may bleed, hookworm infestation.

Any foreign substance reaching the blood appears to be more or less toxic; the harm is prevented by vitamin C, but the vitamin itself is destroyed in the process, states Adelle Davis in *Let's Eat Right to Keep Fit*.

"For example," she says, "every drug apparently destroys vitamin C in the body. It has been found that a single tablet of any one of several drugs widely used and considered harmless can continue to destroy vitamin C in the body for three weeks or longer after the drug is taken. Aspirin, which frequently causes internal hemorrhages, can be dangerous unless our diets contain enough vitamin C to detoxify it."

In *Let's Get Well*, Adelle Davis reports that aspirin interferes with digestion, the formation of body starch, the production of tissue proteins, and the ability of the cells to absorb sugar; it slows the clotting of blood, increases the need for oxygen and for every known nutrient, and accelerates the urinary losses of calcium, potassium, vitamin C and all the B vitamins.

"Many cases of severe (aspirin) toxicity have been reported, causing ulcers, loss of hearing and ringing, roaring and hissing sounds in the ears, especially among persons given the 'full aspirin treatment' for arthritis.

"It is because of its toxicity that aspirin is given for arthritis," she continues. "One doctor, an authority on stress, colorfully describes the treatment as 'a kick in the pants for the tired adrenals,' forcing them to produce a little more cortisone. In the process, however, aspirin depletes these glands of vitamin C and pantothenic acid, causing them to hemorrhage, and unless the diet is unusually adequate, to become exhausted. Many drugs similarly induce stress, and exhaust the pituitary and adrenals."

Since aspirin can irritate the stomach lining, it should always be taken after meals or with milk, says Jane Henry Stolten, R.N., in *Home Care*. She adds that aspirin increases perspiration, so care should be taken to prevent exposure to chill. It is also helpful to crush the tablet and take it in fruit juice or milk, rather than whole.

Aspirin—acetylsalicylic acid—is a most remarkable chemical from the standpoint of its physiological effects and is the best known and most widely used nonbiological weapon, reports Dr. Roger J. Williams in *Nutrition Against Disease*. People buy it along with their groceries, and it is consumed in the U.S. at the rate of about 15 tons a day, he says. To damn aspirin is almost like damning motherhood, but in spite of its palliative effects it must be classed as an essentially "bad" weapon when it is used consistently to cover up trouble which needs more fundamental attention, he adds.

"Aspirin is, for example, used extensively and continuously in the treatment of arthritis. Arthritis is obviously not caused by a lack of aspirin in the body, since aspirin probably never existed on this planet before it was made in the laboratory of the German chemist Gerhardt in 1852," Dr. Williams says.

"By the same token, people who are free from arthritis do not stay this way because they have a self-generated supply of aspirin. Aspirin is a pain-killer, but it is not clear that it is either a remedial or a preventive medicine. It does not produce cures, but by disguising symptoms it may interfere with the task of finding cures."

WHAT ABOUT ASPIRIN?

Dr. Carlton Fredericks, writing in *Psycho-Nutrition*, reports that allergy to aspirin is so common that painkillers not based on salicylic acid have won a considerable market; but few consumers realize that this chemical is a natural constituent of such foods as apricots, prunes, peaches, plums, raspberries, grapes, oranges, cucumbers and tomatoes.

"Helpful guidance in avoiding such foods when they are disturbing to those allergic to aspirin, as well as aid in identifying other drugs and chemicals which are potentially troublemakers for the sensitive, may be obtained from the Allergy Foundation of Lancaster County, Box 1424, Lancaster, Pa. 17604."

Accidental aspirin poisonings among young children were a major factor in the adoption of a new Federal law on December 30, 1970—the Poison Prevention Packaging Act—reported *The New York Times*, August 8, 1976.

Government data since then show that aspirin poisonings and fatalities have dropped, but the totals involved are small, the *Times* said. The Federal Consumer Product Safety Commission in Washington, D.C., reports that 46 children under the age of 5 died in 1972 from swallowing aspirin. In 1974, there were 24 deaths.

The *Times* quotes the National Clearinghouse for Poison Control Centers in Bethesda, Maryland as showing that 8,146 children were poisoned by aspirin in 1972; in 1974, 4,837.

More than one-quarter of a group of children with chronic asthma were demonstrated to have an intolerance to aspirin by a small study done at the University of California at Los Angeles, according to *Medical Tribune*, January 22, 1975.

Dr. Gary Rachelefsky suggested that intolerant patients may fail to make an association between ingestion of aspirin or an aspirin compound and a provoked or intensified asthma attack because of the delayed reaction.

"Also ... many compounds contain aspirin or other compounds known to precipitate asthma in aspirin sensitive patients, unknown to the patient. In this latter group (Dr. Rachelefsky) included indomethacin, mefanamic acid, tartrazine (a yellow coloring material used in soft drinks), canned vegetables and some medications," *Medical Tribune* said.

Aspirin can be very dangerous to the pregnant woman, according to an article, "Aspirin In Pregnancy—Dose of Trouble?" in the October 6, 1975 issue of *Medical World News*. Based on their research in Australia, Drs. Edith Collins and Gillian Turner said that women who ingest aspirin and salicylate-based pick-me-ups "risk increased incidence of anemia, ante- and post-partum hemorrhage, prolonged gestation, complicated deliveries, and loss of their babies through stillbirth or prenatal death."

Medical World News quoted Dr. Reba M. Hill, associate professor of pediatrics at Baylor College of Medicine, Houston, Texas, as saying that aspirin ingestion may well be a problem in the United States, "because aspirin is not respected as a drug. Ask a woman if she takes any drugs, and the answer will be no. Then ask her if she takes aspirin, and the answer is yes."

In a study of drugs taken by pregnant women at St. Lukes Episcopal Hospital, Dr. Hill found that, of 156 women, 60 per cent used an analgesic (pain killer) at least several times a week during pregnancy, and about 40 per cent used an analgesic specifically containing aspirin just as often. Salicylate levels can be identified in 40 per cent to 50 per cent of newborn infants, Dr. Hill told *Medical World News*.

"Normally one of the safest of all drugs, aspirin can turn on its user with deadly effect (it kills 100 children or so every year, along with uncounted adults and adolescents).

WHAT ABOUT ASPIRIN?

And while many millions take it safely, two persons in every 1,000 will be hypersensitive and get a violent, sometimes even fatal reaction, often totally without warning and even after having been comfortable with the drug earlier; 5 per cent of people will get heartburn even from a single tablet; and almost three-quarters of those taking aspirin will lose a half to a full teaspoonful of blood from the drug," states Dr. Arthur S. Freese in *Aspirin and Your Health* (Pyramid Books, New York, 1974).

And so we see that aspirin, taken in large amounts, can be very harmful. It affects many organs of the body, such as the brain, heart, kidney and it can have a number of metabolic effects. It can cause ulcers, internal bleeding, stomach upsets, heartburn, allergy, anemia, etc.

On the other side of the ledger, many victims of arthritis find that aspirin is the only thing that can give them relief. Therefore, should you take aspirin, knowing the pros and cons? We cannot make that decision for you. It is up to you and your doctor to decide. Hopefully, at least one of the remedies discussed in this book will alleviate your arthritis symptoms and stop your dependence on aspirin. Obviously, the less aspirin you take the better off you will be.

CHAPTER 29

Systemic Lupus Erythematosus

SYSTEMIC LUPUS ERYTHEMATOSUS (SLE, LE or Lupus) is a chronic inflammatory disease of the connective tissues of the body. Connective tissues are made up of collagen and a glue-like material called *group substance*. SLE is called a collagen disease because these are the tissues which are involved. Other diseases of these same parts of the body are rheumatic fever and rheumatoid arthritis.

According to a pamphlet published by L-E-Anon or Leanon—Lupus Erythematosus Club—the cause of SLE is still unknown, but specialists in general believe that it is a disorder of the body's production of antibodies which are substances used in the body's defense against bacteria and other "invaders" of body cells. The result is that the victim of SLE becomes allergic to some part of his or her own tissues. Some researchers think, instead, that SLE may be caused by viruses.

SLE can strike anyone, but mostly it is a disease of young women. In fact, 85 per cent of SLE victims are in that age group. Symptoms include: pain in the chest, stomach, muscles or joints, muscular weakness, fluid accumulations in feet, ankles, joints or chest and irregular menstrual periods. There may be low grade fever, chills and malaise. In another kind of lupus (Discoid lupus), there is a red scaling rash, usually on the face, ears or chest. This may be very sensitive to sunlight and may become worse after exposure to the sun.

A young Texas woman, Betty Hull, who established Leanon, has the disease herself and has worked out what we think is an excellent dietary program for herself.

She says, in the April, 1978 issue of her interesting and hopeful newsletter that she takes, every day, 10,000 International Units of vitamin A and a vitamin B complex which includes 50 milligrams of each of the B vitamins. We assume that she means that these capsules contain 50 milligrams of those B vitamins usually measured in milligrams and 50 micrograms of those which are measured in micrograms. Betty Hull takes more of these when she is under stress. In addition, she takes 100 milligrams a day of the B vitamin called PABA (para-amino-benzoic acid) and 500 milligrams of the B vitamin pantothenic acid. She says, of pantothenic acid, that she takes it "for pain." She uses it like aspirin, as needed. It also "fixed" her problem of burning feet, she says.

She takes choline, another B vitamin and pyridoxine (B6) for alleviating fluid accumulations, and stiffness, and vitamin B3 (niacin) for her circulation, eyes and emotional stability. She takes usually 1,000 milligrams of vitamin C daily. When she is under stress or threatened with infections, she takes 4,000 milligrams of crystalline vitamin C several times a day. She takes 800 units of Vitamin D daily and 400 International Units of vitamin E. If she foresees health problems, she increases the vitamin E.

Of minerals she takes two bone meal tablets and two dolomite tablets with meals. The bone meal has calcium and phosphorus. The dolomite has calcium and magnesium. And she takes one all-around mineral tablet daily which contains many other minerals and trace minerals.

She also uses, from time to time, other supplements like garlic, herb teas, lecithin, brewers yeast, kelp, desiccated liver, wheat germ and so on.

She says, "I eat a plain, good, fresh food diet, trying to avoid canned goods, instant foods or artificial sweeteners or any food not fresh. No sugar or sweets. Instead of chocolate I use carob; instead of sugar I use honey but even avoid much of that. Health stores have carob, a naturally sweet chocolate (like) powder that is very good. No white bread, cokes, diet drinks, etc. I feel that changing from tap water to bottled distilled water has been very helpful to me. With the news today about our water supplies, I feel it was a good choice for me and my family."

There is much more in Mrs. Hull's newsletter that would be of great interest to people with lupus and their families. Through it all there is a note of good cheer with many letters from members throughout the world who have lupus and write in with helpful practical hints and accounts of their own progress. There is usually also some information about those drugs most prescribed for lupus patients, their benefits and risks.

You can get in touch with Leanon at this address: Mrs. Betty Hull, P.O. Box 10243, Corpus Christi, Texas 78410.

Here is a list of books available on lupus. If someone in your family or circle of friends is suffering from this disorder, these may be very helpful. They are available postpaid from the S.L.E. Foundation of America, Inc., 95 Madison Avenue, Room 1402, New York City, N. Y. 10016.

Living with S.L.E., by Wallace V. Epstein, M.D., and Gina Clewley, M.S.W., a handbook for the SLE patient, $3.35.

Lupus and You—A Guide for Patients, by the St. Louis Medical Center Research Foundation, $1.50.

Primer on Lupus Erythematosus, by John R. Haserick,

M.D., and Robert Kilburn, M.D., $2.50.

The Sun Is My Enemy, by Henrietta Aladjem, one woman's victory over Lupus, $5.50.

Lupus, the Body Against Itself, by Sheldon Paul Blau, M.D., $6.45.

CHAPTER 30

Exercises for Arthritics

"ON A COLD February morning, 57-year-old Esther Gonzalez begins a weekly ritual of situps, leg lifts and deep knee bends. After the warmup, she and 23 other members of her exercise class proceed to such activities as floor hockey, trampoline maneuvers and gymnastics," wrote Jody Brott Lampert in *The New York Times,* March 1, 1978.

Mrs. Lampert was discussing an exercise class for the elderly sponsored by the Chicago Park District. Ages of the participants range from 65 to 82. Mrs. Lampert quoted C. Carson Conrad, Executive Director of the President's Council on Physical Fitness and Sports, Washington, D.C., as saying that, in the last three years, fitness classes for the elderly have been started in nearly every major American city.

Mr. Conrad, 66, told Mrs. Lampert that in 1977 he conducted workshops on fitness for the elderly in 12 states and 32 counties or cities, with more than 140,000 volunteer leaders participating.

He noted that osteoarthritis is typical of most people over the age of 50. "But you can't give in to it—you just have to stretch and stretch," he said. "By actually being involved in activities that stretch the ligaments and supporting tissue, the senior citizens find they are able to maintain a more upright posture and have better muscular strength to maintain the skeletal structure."

He added, "People really don't stoop because they're old. They're old because they stoop."

The Chicago park program was designed by Jane Jurew, who has been with the parks district for 25 years. Mrs. Jurew carefully monitors the temperature of the gym floor to insure that none of her charges get chilled. And she also checks for overexertion.

"I watch for puffiness or redness in the face," she said. "I know their coloring, their ways, their breathing. If anything changes in the slightest, I know it."

So far there have been no serious injuries or ill effects from the exercise, Mrs. Jurew said.

Irene Tezky, one of the participants, who admitted that she was "60 plus," reported that, before starting the exercise class, she could not wash her windows because of arthritis. Now she cleans them from the top step of a ladder. Another exerciser, 76-year-old Maria Zimmerman, pointed to where she had pains before she began exercising regularly. "Now it hurts no more," she said.

As we have reported in this book, folk remedies abound for treating arthritis. Some of these remedies involve immobilizing the injured joints. Now it seems that this may be just about the worst thing one can do in treating arthritis, for it seems that exercise is one of the most important and beneficial therapies for this painful disorder.

"Go home and exercise," doctors say to patients with arthritis. Such instruction is as valid as saying to a diabetic, "Go home and eat," according to Dr. Nila Kirkpatrick Covalt, writing in the *Southern Medical Journal* for July 1962. The *way* arthritics exercise is the important thing, she believes. So, for the arthritic, getting the right exercises for him as an individual and doing them faithfully every day may mean the difference between reasonably good health and the life of a deformed and helpless cripple.

Dr. Covalt says further that drugs for arthritis are in the same category as crutches and splints—just aids to help the patient get along a bit better—nothing more. Cortisone was announced as the miracle drug. It relieves pain, she says, but it also produces a whole new group of symptoms never before seen. It has not prevented deformities or stiff joints.

Stiffening joints involve many different muscles. A knowledge of these muscles and their relationship to one another is essential for knowing what exercises to do or what massage and manipulation by someone else will be helpful. This is the reason why professional therapists do a much better job than a member of one's family, who simply wants to help, but may do harm instead.

Arthritics who are not given instructions on how to exercise tend to choose "flexion" exercises. That is, they bend their elbows and knees and clench their hands. If their hands are stiff, they squeeze rubber balls. Dr. Covalt says that the muscles that govern this bending process are much stronger than the muscles that pull the other way. Since most stiff joints are already bent, bending them still further is the worst thing you can do. Instead, they should be exercised in other ways to strengthen the muscles that pull against the "bending" muscles.

If shoulders and back are stiff, the best way to exercise them is to move the arms away from the body—to the side. And to lie face down on a bed for stretching the back. Sitting for long hours keeps the knees and hips bent, thereby making the bad joints which are already bent worse.

Says Dr. Covalt: "There is no substitute for active

exercise for the arthritic, no matter what treatment he receives that may alleviate his pain. . . . Active exercise must be continued with all muscles that are already weak or will weaken. . . . Active exercise needs to be done daily and usually twice a day. No exercise is ever done more than 10 times in any exercise period."

Massage is passive exercise. And apparently it is done incorrectly much more often than correctly. The patient himself mistakenly massages his painful joints, says Dr. Covalt. This is an almost automatic gesture, especially with painful hands and wrists. Massaging over a painful joint merely increases the inflammation there. Professional therapists know, she says, that massage should never be given *over* a joint. Massage does not improve the condition of the muscles, nor prevent their atrophy. It does improve circulation, but active exercise by the patient does this even more effectively.

She says that there is no doubt that some arthritics feel better if they have scientific massage. Massage of the back is probably most helpful. It may relax the patient and make him less tense. He and the therapist should discuss the effects they are getting with massage and then come to a decision as to whether they are worth the time and money expended.

The arthritic is handicapped so far as daily living is concerned. Does he need someone—a nurse perhaps—to dress him, feed him, hand him things, run and fetch for him? Dr. Covalt believes firmly that the basic rule of rehabilitation is to *never do for a patient what he can do for himself*. He may need more time than a healthy person, but he must be encouraged to "do for himself" or he will surely become helpless. Such a condition is harmful so far as muscles and joints are concerned. It is perhaps even more harmful to the patient's mental state. To know that he is dependent is psychologically very disturbing.

Dr. Covalt recommends a booklet available from the Public Health Service, in collaboration with the Arthritis and Rheumatism Foundation. It is called *Strike Back at Arthritis*. The booklet was available from the Superintendent of Documents, Washington, D.C. 20502, but it is now out of print.

However, the booklet has been revised by The Arthritis Foundation, under the title of *Home Care Programs in Arthritis—a Manual for Patients*. It is free for the asking. The Arthritis Foundation chapter in your area probably has a copy. You can find their address in your phone book. The booklet is intended for physicians to give to their arthritic patients. At the same time they can earmark certain exercises for the patient and make certain he understands how to do them. Some sample exercises are shown with this chapter.

The very readable, well-designed and well-illustrated book describes exercises to be done by the patient himself, along with "assisted" exercises to be done with a therapist or a "helper." There is a section on posture—how to lie in bed, how to sit, how to stand, how to walk. There are instructions for applying heat and a final section on self-help devices such as utensils for those whose hands are badly crippled with arthritis.

Dr. Currier McEwen of New York University Medical Center, writing in *Archives of Environmental Health*, May 1962, tells us that the internist or general practitioner sometimes fails to realize the tremendous importance of orthopedic procedures, like exercise, massage and so forth, whereas the medical man who specializes in orthopedics sometimes does not appreciate fully that arthritis is a generalized, systemic disease. That is, it afflicts the entire patient and all of him must be treated—not just the sore, inflamed joints.

Faced with a disease as painful, baffling and mysterious

as arthritis, most of us seek whatever help the medical profession can give us and, when we discover how limited are their resources, we ask ourselves, "What can I do for myself? Surely there must be some way I can lick this thing."

That was what happened to Dvera Berson, who became arthritic at 54 and spent the next five and a half years going through all the therapy medical science knows of, only to find that she was never free from excruciating pain, that she had to wear braces and collars, her hands were deformed and crippled, and she had taken all the drugs it was safe to take.

She's a very determined and resourceful woman. A vacation in Florida showed her that she could move her aching joints much more easily under water. Back home, she joined a health club and spent several hours every day in their pool. Gradually, as she developed underwater exercises for this and that part of her body, she found that the pain was lessening.

Eventually she could report, "As of this writing, I have absolutely no pain. I can proudly walk with my head up. I don't wear a cervical collar or use a back support or do any traction. I don't take drugs or visit doctors for arthritis. My fingers are no longer deformed."

She is not cured of arthritis. If she goes off her exercise program for even a month, pain and stiffness begin to return. But as long as she continues her regular exercise program, she can keep the pain and stiffness at bay. She must take a bus to the indoor swimming pool. Waiting for the bus is inconvenient and unpleasant, especially in winter. But the benefits are well worth every inconvenience.

In her book on the subject (*Pain-Free Arthritis*, published by Simon and Schuster, 1230 Avenue of the Americas, New York City 10020, $6.95), Dvera Berson and her co-author, Sander Roy, start with the easiest exercises and show you exactly how and what to do, with very clear sketches to help out. They progress through intermediate to advanced exercises, giving some suggestions for exercising at home in the tub and some hints for paraphernalia you may find helpful in the swimming pool.

This is a small book of less than 100 pages. Its author wastes no time describing what arthritis is and how it affects you. She gets right into the story of her successful exercise program. Throughout she stresses the fact that you must be determined and persevering. This is no program you can try for a couple of weeks and then abandon. It is a program which can, she says, keep you in good health without pain or crippling for the rest of your life, if you stick with it. But you must stick with it.

We're quite ready to believe she's right. Diet is not mentioned in these pages. As you know by now, we believe that what you eat and do not eat has a great deal to do with joint diseases. If Ms. Berson can get these results without even making any changes in her diet, then someone who eats with great care and knowledge of good nutrition can probably get even better results. We think it's well worth trying. Daily exercises are bound to help prevent and treat many other devastating diseases, as well, such as heart and circulatory ones, so this should be an added benefit.

While on the peripheral area of exercise, we can report that Dr. Richard Rogal of the Ranchos Los Amigos Hospital in Los Angeles, California, told a meeting of the American Rheumatism Association in New Orleans, Louisiana that three-fourths of all patients with rheumatoid arthritis are capable of leading satisfactory sex lives. Dr. Rogal urged physicians to explain more specifically how each individual can surmount his or her problem.

"Arthritics have the same need to be loved physically and emotionally as the rest of humanity," Dr. Rogal is quoted as saying in *Medical Tribune*, July 23, 1975. "There is a temptation for the practitioner who is uncomfortable about discussing sex just to hand out the pamphlets. But more guidance is required."

Dr. Rogal believes that only about one-fourth of arthritis patients have physical handicaps severe enough to rule out sexual acts completely.

"Patients with sex problems often question their value as mates, mothers, fathers, breadwinners and homemakers," he continued. "Young people are especially vulnerable. They start to wonder whether anybody will ever love them the way they are."

In the previously mentioned booklet, *Home Care Programs in Arthritis—A Manual for Patients*, The Arthritis Foundation describes the various canes and crutches for those who need them and offers suggestions for using them. For example, your "crutch gait" or the gait at which you walk can determine your stability and safety while moving about.

Arthritis frequently affects the feet, so there are tips on selecting the right kind of shoes. For feet that are badly deformed or painful, your physician may recommend specially made shoes.

There are a variety of self-help devices available for those who already have arthritis. These include: long-handled combs, wash cloth mitt with soap pocket, large-handled cup, long-handled reaching tongs, built-up pencil, long-handled shoe horn, built-up spoon, long-handled fork, long-handled tooth brush, button aid, jar opener, raised toilet seat, chair on blocks, etc.

There are suggestions for rearranging your kitchen for easy mobility; how to select a cart or wheeled table for moving things around your house or apartment; tips on selecting furniture; devices for use in the bathroom; selecting a wheelchair, etc.

What about hot and cold applications? Neither will

improve your arthritis but they may give you temporary relief from aches and pains, the booklet says. The Arthritis Foundation also makes these recommendations:

1. Cold compresses or an ice bag (or ice cubes in a plastic bag wrapped in a towel) will have a numbing effect and give some relief from pain where they are applied.

2. Heat will relax muscle spasm. Heat is especially helpful when used just before doing exercises. Warming the muscles tends to relax them and may make the exercises more efficient.

3. Various types of heat may be used . . . such as heat lamps, heating pads, warm compresses, tub baths, paraffin baths.

4. A daily tub bath in warm water is often the most effective way to apply heat to widely separated joints at the same time. Staying in water that is too hot, however, or even in "comfortably" warm water for over 20 minutes once a day, may be very fatiguing and should be avoided.

5. When you wish to heat only small areas of your body, hot compresses are effective. Use a piece of wool or a towel. It should be soaked in hot water, wrung out thoroughly and put on the painful joint. A sheet of plastic wrapped over the compress will retain the heat longer.

6. A 250-watt infra-red reflector heat bulb (not a sun lamp or ultraviolet light) is effective for heating a single area of the body. It should be kept two or three feet from the skin and used for not longer than one-half hour at a time.

7. Heating pads are convenient but are safe only if in good condition and when properly used. They should be used only on low heat and for short periods of time. *Never* lie on a heating pad and *don't* go to sleep with a heating pad left on your body.

8. Paraffin baths are particularly useful for stiff or inflamed hands and wrists. But don't use paraffin if you

have any open cuts or wounds on your hands.

To prepare a paraffin bath, put four pounds of paraffin wax and two ounces of mineral oil into the upper part of a three quart double boiler (with plenty of water in the

---

POSTURE CHECKLIST

STANDING —Stand straight, head high, shoulders straight, stomach in, hips and knees straight.

WALKING —Walk erect, as in standing position.
—Keep hips and knees straight.
—Let arms swing easily at sides.
—Do not sag or shuffle.

SITTING —Use straight-back arm chair with firm seat.
—Sit with head up, shoulders straight, stomach in.
—Keep feet flat on floor.

IN BED —Lie straight, flat on back.
—Keep knees and hips straight, arms and hands straightened at sides.
—Use board between mattress and bedspring to keep mattress firm.
—If you need a pillow under your head, use a small one.
—Never put a pillow under your knees.

Courtesy "Home Care Programs in Arthritis—a Manual for Patients."

---

bottom section). Heat until the wax is melted. Remove from the heat and allow the wax to cool until a thin white coating appears on top. It is then ready for use.

When heating paraffin, be extremely careful to keep it away from an open flame. Never melt it in a pot directly over flame; always use a double boiler.

With your fingers slightly separated, dip your hands, one at a time, quickly into and out of the paraffin. Re-dip them seven or eight times, allowing the wax to cool on your hands between dippings. Once you have started to dip, do not move your fingers because the paraffin will crack.

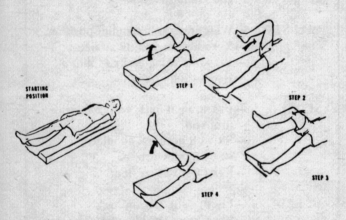

HIP AND KNEE FLEXION AND EXTENSION

Lift your leg, bending it at the knee and at the hip. Continue to move the leg, bringing the knee toward your chest so that the hip and knee are bent as far as they will go. (Keep other leg flat on the bed). Lower your leg, then straighten the knee by lifting the foot upward. Return to the starting position, rest, then repeat the exercise.

Have someone wrap your hands in a plastic bag or paper towel and keep them still for about 20 minutes. The wax will crack and peel off cleanly and can be put back into the boiler for use again when needed. Paraffin may be applied to larger joints with a paint brush.

9. There are still other methods of applying heat. Discuss them with your doctor or therapist.

10. Whatever the type of heat, take care to avoid burns.

11. And remember that no form of heat has any magical or curative properties. It is used to relieve pain and soreness, and that's all it can do.

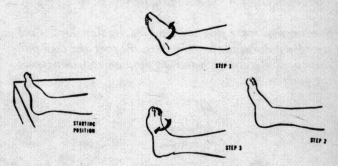

FOOT INVERSION AND EVERSION

Starting position: Lying on your back, leg straight, 1.   Turn your foot in so that the sole faces toward the other foot. 2.   Return to the starting position. 3.   Turn your foot out so that the sole faces away from the other foot. Return to starting position and repeat.

Exercises and drawings courtesy of *Strike Back at Arthritis.*

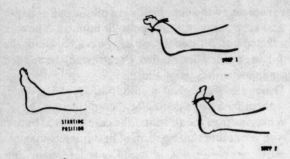

TOE FLEXION AND EXTENSION

Starting position: Lying on your back, leg straight, 1. Curl the toes downward. 2. Straighten the toes and then pull them back. Return to the starting position, rest, then repeat the exercise.

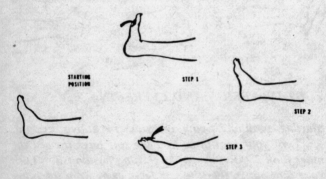

ANKLE DORSI AND PLANTAR FLEXION

Starting position: Lying on your back, leg straight, foot relaxed. 1. Keep the leg straight. Bend your ankle, pointing your toes toward you. 2. Relax your foot. 3. Bend your ankle, pointing your toes away from you. Rest, then repeat the exercise.

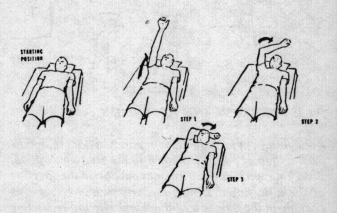

SHOULDER FLEXION

Keep your elbow straight and lift your arm until your hand points to the ceiling. Continue to move the arm back until it rests on the bed next to your head. The arm may be bent at the elbow if the headboard of the bed will not permit the arm to be carried all the way back. Return to the starting position, rest, then repeat the exercise.

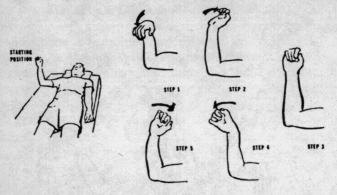

WRIST FLEXION AND EXTENSION

Bend your wrist forward as far as possible; bend your wrist back as far as possible. Return to the starting position. Bend your wrist sidewise as far as possible in the direction of the little finger. Bend your wrist sidewise as far as possible in the direction of the thumb. Return to starting position, rest, then repeat the exercise.

EXERCISES FOR ARTHRITICS

The Need to Work with Your Hands

Your hands and arms are most important in your being able to do things for yourself, to care for yourself. Exercises 1 through 6 will help you to keep your hands and arms functional.

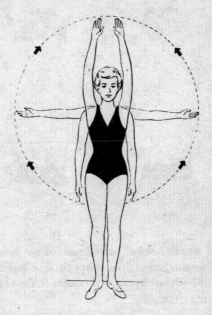

Exercise 1:

Raise your arms as high as you can over your head, keeping your elbows straight. Then swing your arms out and down to your sides. Swing your arms in as big a circle as possible. This exercise is best done when standing but it can also be performed while sitting or lying. Repeat three to six times.

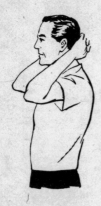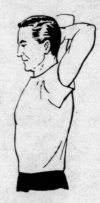

Exercise 2:

Place your hands behind your head. Move your elbows back as far as you can. As you move your elbows back, pull your chin in and move your head back. Return to starting position and repeat.

Drawings beginning on page 213 courtesy of *Home Care Programs in Arthritis—a Manual for Patients.*

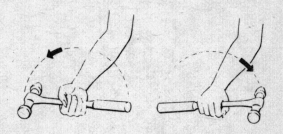

Exercise 3:

Grasp the handle of a medium-weight hammer firmly near its head. Keep your upper arm by your side and bend your arm at the elbow to a right angle. Turn your wrist from left to right and back so that the hammer turns out and in. Let the weight of the hammer swing your hand over as far as possible each time. Repeat with the other hand. Repeat three to six times with each hand. As you improve, shift your grip further toward the end of the handle so that the weight of the hammer makes you work harder.

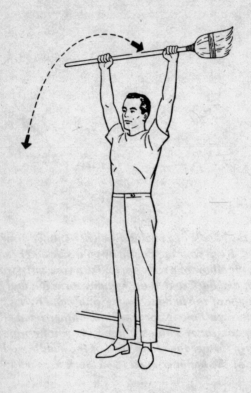

Exercise 4A:

Stand with your back against a wall with your heels, buttocks, shoulder blades and head touching it. Grasp a broomstick or cane in both hands and raise it as high above your head as possible, keeping your elbows as straight as you can. Then lower your arms. Repeat.

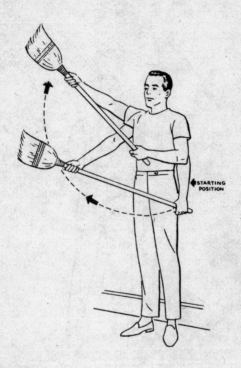

STARTING POSITION

Exercise 4B:

Stand against a wall, as in 4A. With your arms straight down, move your hands two to three feet apart on the stick. Swing the stick up to the right (it helps to think of pushing with your left hand), keeping your right elbow straight and against the wall if possible. Return to the starting position and swing the stick up to the left in the same way, keeping your left elbow straight. Repeat.

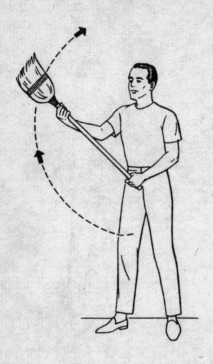

Exercise 4C:

Grab the stick as shown and push it up as if you were shoveling snow over your right shoulder. Change your grip and repeat the motion over your left shoulder. Repeat.

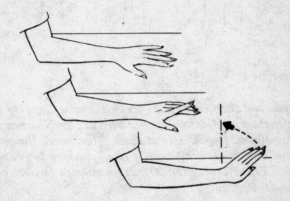

Exercise 5:

Place your hand flat on a table or, if you are in bed, flat on your stomach. If you can't get your hand completely flat, keep trying, and do the exercise anyway. First, spread your fingers apart, keeping them as straight as possible. Then lift your index finger. Now lift all your fingers, including the thumb, keeping your palm pressed down. Then lift your fingers, the thumb and your hand as far as possible, keeping your forearm on the table and bending your wrist up as far as you can.

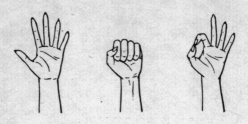

Exercise 6:

Open and close your hands, spreading your fingers as you open them, and making as tight a fist as possible when you close them. Repeat several times. Then touch the tip of your thumb to each finger in turn, pinching firmly each time. Try to form a letter "O" at each attempt. Do with both hands. Repeat.

The Need to Move About

Your legs must have enough strength and flexibility to get you up and carry you from place to place. Walking is good exercise, provided the joints of your knees or ankles are not swollen, painful, or stiff. If they are, then limit your standing and walking but maintain strength and joint motion with Exercises 7 through 10.

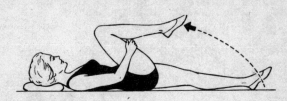

Exercise 7:

Lie on your back. Bend your right knee up toward your chest. Bend both your knee and hip as far as possible. Use your hands to pull your knee toward you if necessary. Then lower your leg slowly, straightening your knee as you do. Repeat the exercise with your left leg. Repeat three to six times with each leg.

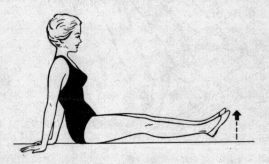

Exercise 8:

Sit as shown or lie flat on your back with your legs straight. Push your thighs down against the bed and lift your heels up about one inch. This will tighten and straighten your knees. If you cannot straighten your knees, put a rolled towel under them, and then push your knees down against the towel and lift your heels as much as you can. Repeat.

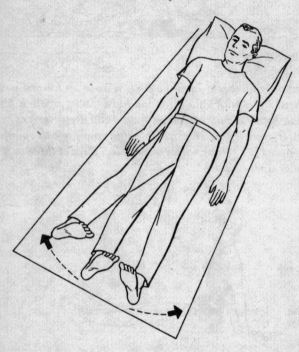

Exercise 9:

Lie flat on your back, legs straight and about six inches apart. Point the toes together. First, move the right leg out to the side and return, then the left leg out and return, still keeping your toes pointing together. Repeat.

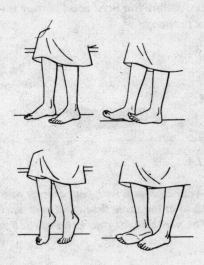

Exercise 10:

Sit in a chair with your feet flat on the floor. First, raise your toes as high as you can while keeping the heels down. Then keep your toes down and lift your heels as high as possible. Next, starting with your feet flat on the floor, lift the inside of each foot and roll the weight over on the outside of the foot. Keep your toes curled down if possible. Repeat.

ARTHRITIS

The Need to Maintain Good
Posture and Breathing Habits

Posture exercises and breathing exercises (Exercises 11 through 13) go hand in hand. A series of ten very deep breaths is one of the best posture exercises you can do. One of the major reasons you need good posture is so that you can breathe properly.

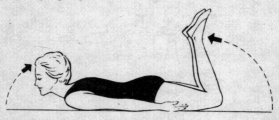

Exercise 11A:

Lie flat on your stomach, with your arms at your sides. Lift your head and at the same time bend your knees as far as possible. You may also lift your knees a little if you are able to.

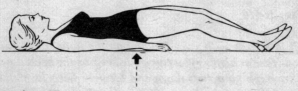

Exercise 11B:

If you cannot lie flat on your stomach, substitute this exercise: Lie flat on your back, with your legs straight, push your heels and shoulders down against the bed and lift your buttocks off the bed. Hold the position for a few seconds. Repeat.

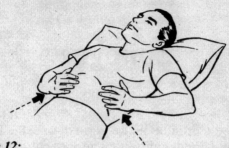

Exercise 12:

Lie flat on your back with your hands on the sides of your chest. Now breathe in deeply and push your ribs out against your hands. Hold a moment, then breathe out. Be sure to take a breath deep enough to push the ribs outward. Repeat.

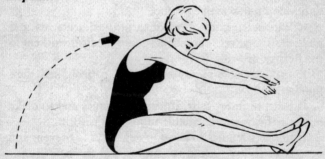

Exercise 13:

Lie on your back with your knees as straight as possible. First, lift your head so that your chin is on your chest. Then come to a sitting position, reaching with your hands toward your toes. Lie back down and repeat. However, if you have low back problems, this exercise should be done with your knees bent enough so that your feet are flat on the floor (or other surface).

Epilogue

A YEAR AGO or so before we began to write this book we wrote to a number of sources of material—or what we innocently thought might be sources of material—for example, the Arthritis Foundation, a nation-wide tax-free foundation which collects vast sums of money every year in order to perform the following functions, according to their own literature:

It supports research to discover the cause of arthritis and to develop a preventive or cure.

It finances training for young medical scientists and physicians; and seeks to attract more medical workers to the field of arthritis.

It expands community services to patients and their families.

It seeks to improve treatment techniques and to make better arthritis care available to all who need it.

It finances studies to develop new ways to prevent and correct disability,... and to develop and test new drugs.

It informs doctors and patients of the latest development in arthritis.

We wrote also to the National Institutes of Health, a federal bureau supported entirely by taxpayers' money. One of the institutes is called the National Institute of Arthritis, Metabolism and Digestive Diseases. That was where we innocently expected to get lots of material to help us in writing this book. We had no answer or any acknowledgement from the National Institute of Arthritis,

Metabolism and Digestive Diseases, for a long, long time, although we kept writing, making the same request time after time.

Finally, we wrote to our congressman, asking him to see if he could pry this information out of this gigantic bureaucracy. Very shortly, we received from the Institute a clutch of leaflets from *The Arthritis Foundation*—the very same things we had already received from the Foundation. We wrote again to the Institute, explaining that we had already contacted the Foundation, had received all the material they had available. Is it possible, we asked, that the vast National Institute of Arthritis, Metabolism and Digestive Diseases has nothing of its own in the way of information to offer a taxpayer whose money supports all of the Institute's activities? We pointed out that there are 74 highly paid professional men working at the NIH. What are they doing? we asked.

We received another letter from the Office of Scientific and Technical Reports of the National Institute of Arthritis, Metabolism and Digestive Diseases. He apologized for not realizing that we were not just plain people but "Writers" and told us at length that

"The National Institute of Arthritis, Metabolism and Digestive Diseases is not engaged solely in research on arthritis, but also in gastroenterology and nutrition, urology and kidney diseases, diabetes and metabolic disorders, diseases of blood, bone, and skin, the field of orthopedic surgery and disorders of the endocrine glands, among other fields and disciplines. Thus those 74 top scientists you mentioned as working in the arthritis disorders are actually engaged in other types of research. We do have three or four investigators here at NIH engaged in full-time clinical and basic studies in arthritis. The overwhelming mass of our arthritis research, of course, is performed by grant-supported scientists at various medical centers and universities across the country."

He then went on to tell us how we might be able to get information from the National Library of Medicine "through which all research advances, not just that supported or performed by the NIAMDD, are reported." He enclosed several meaningless leaflets from The National Commission on Arthritis and Related Musculo-skeletal Diseases and a report entitled *Arthritis Out of the Maze, Volume I, The Arthritis Plan.* This is a report from a group of 20 people, only two of whom are based at the NIAMDD. The report went to the President of the United States Senate and the Speaker of the House on April 20, 1976.

It proposes, in essence, a plan for "productive action" to "respond to the multifaceted challenge" of about 10.3 per cent of the American population who suffer from one or another of the arthritic diseases—about 22 million of them. The Commission which produced this 186-page report was established by the National Arthritis Act signed into law in January, 1975.

The same Act went on to propose a number of other activities such as provision for financial grants for many kinds of community activity, establishment of an arthritis data bank to collect pertinent material, the development of arthritis centers for research, diagnosis, treatment, etc etc, the establishment of an Associate Director in the NIAMDD to be in charge of just arthritis.

Fifteen other provisions were laid out, all of them very lofty, very grandiose, very inspiring, *very expensive.* In one of these provisions we found the word "prevention" and— wonder of wonders—we found the word "nutrition"—two words that almost never appear in anything released by the federal government on the subject of health. We were encouraged by these two words into thinking that perhaps somewhere in that vast bureaucracy in Foggy Bottom somebody still thought that it might be possible—just might be possible—to do some research on ways to *prevent* arthritis and, God willing, might be able to contemplate even trying to prevent arthritis by using good *nutrition* as the chief tool. After all, those two words "prevention" and "nutrition" *had* appeared in the report.

We realized that this was probably a vain hope, since all of the official literature from the government and from The Arthritis Foundation states flatly, very flatly, that diet in any form has absolutely nothing to do with arthritis or any of the diseases in this category. Nothing, understand. Nothing. And it's only cranks, faddists and health nuts who go on talking about nutrition and diet as if they had anything at all to do with human health! The general public must beware of these greedy quacks!

Encouraged by mention of the two words nutrition and prevention, we decided to try the Public Health Service. In April 1966 they had published a rather informative little book called *Arthritis Source Book, Public Health Service Publication No. 1431*. We wrote a polite letter to the Public Health Service inquiring if, by chance, they had updated this book, since we were writing on arthritis and wanted the latest material. If they had updated it, we said, could they tell us what the updated version is called, where it is available and how much it costs.

That letter went out the middle of August, 1977. Not unexpectedly, we heard nothing from the Public Health Service. We are used to receiving no reply from any government bureau unless we enlist the help of our congressman to pry the answer out of them. Several months went by and we wrote several more times to the Public Health Service. It was like dropping the letter into a bottomless pit. Maybe, we decided, the Public Health Service *is* a bottomless pit. Maybe there's nothing else there but a bottomless pit and an address.

For two weeks we wrote every day to the Public Health

Service, sending them a copy of our original letter and reminding them how long it had gone unanswered. They did not reply. We finally wrote our congressman and asked him to pry an answer out of the Public Health Service if, indeed, the Public Health Service was still in existence.

Several days later we received a large envelope from the Public Health Service. Inside it—can you guess? You're right—another copy of the booklet *Arthritis: Out of the Maze, Volume I, The Arthritis Plan,* along with a printed slip thanking us for our request.

On several later occasions we received in the mail other copies of the booklet *Arthritis: Out of the Maze, Volume I, The Arthritis Plan.* We have a pile of them now, and nothing—absolutely nothing else from the vast federal health bureaucracy in Washington. Oh, yes, there's a little 15-page leaflet called *How to Cope With Arthritis* which tells you that there is nothing you can do for arthritis except to see your doctor and do exactly what he or she says.

So, friends, don't look to the federal government or any branch of the federal government to give you any help on your problems with arthritis. They have available to spend every year as much as 39 million dollars of your tax money. This is what you get out of it. After some 50 years or so of shuffling around, mumbling to one another and giving and getting financial grants, that branch of the federal government charged with protecting and maintaining your health has precisely *nothing* to offer the 22 million people in this country who have arthritis in one form or another. Nothing.

From time to time in this book we have used material from the *Arthritis Source Book* and *Arthritis: Out of the Maze,* since there is no other source for this kind of material except for the federal government.

We have also used material that we personally have gathered at great cost in time, money and energy over the past 25 years or so. This material deals, for the most part, with what *you* and you alone *can* do to help prevent arthritis and to do whatever you can to ease the pain and prevent further pain and destruction of body tissues.

We have combed this material out of hundreds of scientific and medical publications. Most of it deals with nutritional remedies. We think it is helpful. We have many testimonials from people who have tried one or another, or several, or many of these suggested therapies and preventive methods and have found them sound and helpful. That is why we are putting them into this book.

All this material is available to anyone who chooses to seek it out—including the high-salaried medical men and administrators in the Public Health Service, the National Institute of Health and the medical establishment. They have not only not sought it out, they have insisted that it does not exist. With one voice, they tell you that what you eat and drink has nothing to do with your health or with your susceptibility to arthritis. We think, after you have read this book, you may disagree with that flat dictum.

We do not know why the medical establishment and the people who serve them, chiefly in Washington bureaus, refuse to admit that such information exists and can be used to good purpose to prevent illness and maintain good health. You must ask *them* why.

We have a number of unconfirmed suspicions. It seems to us that this reluctance to permit any American to do anything to maintain his or her own health and prevent chronic diseases may have something to do with the fact that the medical establishment depends on the detail men of the drug industry for practically all their information on the treatment of disease. There seems to be no other conceivable reason why the medical profession and practically all its associated professional men in every branch of government and every "health" foundation cry as with one voice, "Don't dare to treat yourself for any disease. And, most of all, don't dare to believe that what you put into your mouth in the way of food and drink has anything at all to do with your health".

You are, of course, at liberty to draw your own conclusions as to why there is nothing available from the federal government for a private individual or even a writer on the subject of our most widespread and most agonizingly painful group of diseases. You are also at liberty to scoff at or discard some, most, or all of the material presented in this book. Or you can accept some of it, or all of it as it is presented—in good faith.

It is our belief that the American public has the right to know that there is a great deal of information in standard medical and scientific literature pointing to many steps the average individual *can* take which may prevent arthritis or may lessen its impact on someone who already has the disease. We think you have the right to know this, and we think you are intelligent enough to understand it and to use it or not, as you wish, without any dictums from any foundation or government bureau insisting that you are too uninformed or too inept to do anything for yourself, but must immediately turn yourself over to a physician who will give you a lot of expensive, fatiguing and painful tests and then—very probably, tell you to go home and take some aspirin. Aspirin is the officially recommended treatment for arthritis, the consummation of everything all the vast might of our federal power, money and professional expertise can produce to relieve the agonizing pain and pitiful crippling of arthritis.

The following free leaflets are available from the Arthritis Foundation:

Arthritis in Children.

Systemic Lupus Erythematosus.

The Arthritis Foundation, What It Is and What It Does.
Home Care Programs in Arthritis.
Arthritis, the Basic Facts.
The Truth About Aspirin for Arthritis.
Arthritis in Women.
Arthritis and Social Security Benefits.
Today's Facts About Arthritis.
Rheumatoid Arthritis, a Handbook for Patients.
About Gout.
Osteoarthritis, a Handbook for Patients.
Gout, a Handbook for Patients.

Arthritis—Literature for the patient and the public available from the Arthritis Foundation.

The National Office of the Arthritis Foundation is 3400 Peachtree Rd., N.E., Atlanta, Ga. 30326. There is probably a local chapter in or near your own city. You can find the address in the phone book or ask the National Office of the Arthritis Foundation for the address.

The federal government has one 15-page leaflet saying almost nothing. This is available from the U.S. Department of Health, Education and Welfare, Public Health Service, National Institutes of Health—DHEW publication no. (NIH) 76-1092. *How to Cope With Arthritis.*

Glossary

ACUPUNCTURE: Ancient Chinese technique of using needles to pierce parts of the body to treat disease and relieve pain.

ADRENOCORTICAL HORMONE: Substance manufactured in the natural form, in the adrenal glands. Such hormones are now manufactured synthetically and can be used in the treatment of arthritis.

ANKYLOSING SPONDYLITIS: A chronic, progressive disease of the small joints of the spine, separable from rheumatoid arthritis on genetic, epidemiologic, pathologic, clinical, serologic, and therapeutic grounds; Marie-Strümpell Disease.

ANKYLOSIS: Stiffening and fixation of a joint.

ANTIBODY: A protein produced by the body in response to a foreign substance with the specific capacity to neutralize—and create immunity to—that substance.

ANTIGEN: A substance, usually a protein, capable of provoking the body to make an antibody against it.

ANTI-INFLAMMATORY: Counteracting or suppressing inflammation.

ANTIMICROBIAL: Agent to destroy the action of microorganisms, prevent their development, or their pathogenic action.

ANTIRHEUMATIC: A drug which suppresses symptoms and inflammation in rheumatic diseases.

ARTERITIS: Inflammation of an artery.

ARTHR-, ARTHRO-: Denoting relationship to a joint or joints.

—Source: *Volume I: The Arthritis Plan, National Commission on Arthritis and Related Musculoskeletal Diseases,* Report to the Congress of the United States, April, 1976.

GLOSSARY

ARTHRALGIA: Joint pain.

ARTHRITIS: Inflammation of a joint.

ARTICULAR CARTILAGE: A thin layer of gristle or elastic substance on the surface of bones where they meet to form a joint.

ARTICULATION: A place of union or junction between two or more bones of the skeleton; i.e., joint.

ARTIFICIAL JOINT: An artificial substitute for a malfunctioning joint of the body.

ATROPHY: A wasting of the tissues.

AUTOIMMUNE DISEASE: Condition in which structural and/or functional change is produced by the action of immunologically competent cells or antibodies against normal components of the body.

BACTERIAL ARTHRITIS: Inflammation of a joint or joints caused by bacteria within the joint(s).

BIOFEEDBACK: A technique for controlling emotional states to modify involuntary body functions.

BURSA: Sac or saclike cavity filled with a viscid fluid, situated between a tendon and a bone to facilitate joint motion.

BURSITIS: Acute or chronic inflammation of a bursa.

CALCIFICATION: Process by which organic tissue becomes hardened by a deposit of calcium salts within its substance.

CAPSULAR INFLAMMATION: Inflammation of the membrane structure that envelops an organ, joint, or other structure.

CARTILAGE: The gristle or elastic substance attached to articular bone surfaces.

CHONDROCYTE: A cartilage cell.

CHRONIC DISEASE: A disease of slow progress and long continuance.

COLLAGEN: The main supportive protein of skin, tendon, bone, cartilage, and connective tissue.

ARTHRITIS

COLLAGEN DISEASE: Connective tissue disease.

CONGENITAL DYSPLASIA: A dislocation, present at birth, of the head of the femur and acetabulum. One of the most common causes of hip problems in childhood and subsequent osteoarthritis in later life; congenital dislocation.

CONJUNCTIVITIS: Inflammation of the membrane covering the surface of the eye.

CONNECTIVE TISSUE: The tissues which provide the supportive framework and protective covering of the body and its internal organs. Includes bone, periosteum, cartilage, tendon, tendon sheath, ligament, and fascia.

CONNECTIVE TISSUE DISEASE: One of the conditions characterized by inflammation and widespread changes in connective tissue, esp. collagen tissue, such as rheumatic fever, acute systemic lupus erythematosus, scleroderma, dermatomyositis, rheumatoid arthritis, periateritis nodosa.

CORTICOSTEROID: Substance, usually a hormone, manufactured in the cortex of the adrenal gland. Such substances are also synthesized artificially.

DEGENERATIVE JOINT DISEASE: Osteoarthritis.

DERMATOMYOSITIS: Non suppurative inflammation of the skin, subcutaneous tissue, and underlying muscle.

ENZYME: A protein capable of accelerating or producing by catalytic action some change in a substrate for which it is often specific.

ERYTHEMA NODOSUM: A disorder characterized by the presence of oval or round, slightly raised, hot, painful red nodules on the skin. Arthralgia also occurs.

FASCIA: Band or sheath of connective tissue investing, supporting, or binding together internal organs or parts of the body.

FIBROSIS: Formation of fibrous tissue; fibroid or fibrous degeneration.

GLOSSARY

GOUT: A disease characterized by recurrent episodes of violent arthritis with the presence of urate crystals in the synovial fluid, an excess of uric acid in the blood, and usually, the eventual appearance of tophi in or about the joints, kidneys, and other sites.

GOUTY ARTHRITIS: Arthritis due to gout.

HERNIATED VERTEBRAL DISK DISEASE: Nerve root compression due to protrusion of the disk through the surrounding fibrocartilage.

HORMONE: A chemical substance formed in one organ or part of the body and carried in the blood to another organ or part where it stimulates functional activity or secretion.

IMMUNE RESPONSE: A complex series of cellular events in which specialized lymphocytes are stimulated to respond immunologically to an inciting antigen.

IMMUNITY: A natural or acquired state in which the body is resistant to disease.

IMMUNOLOGICAL DEFECT: An imperfection or failure in the immune response.

IMMUNOSUPPRESSION: Artificial prevention or diminution of the immune response.

IMMUNOSUPPRESSIVE AGENT: An agent which induces immunosuppression.

INFECTIOUS AGENT: A microorganism capable of being transmitted by infection.

INFECTIOUS ARTHRITIS: Arthritis due to infection (e.g., gonococcal, tuberculous).

INFLAMMATION: A localized protective reaction of tissues to injury or destruction, characterized by pain, heat, redness, swelling and loss of function.

JOINT ASPIRATION: Removal of fluid from a joint.

JUVENILE RHEUMATOID ARTHRITIS: A form of arthritis that affects children and may lead to significant disability, morbidity and mortality.

LEGG-PERTHES DISEASE: Arthritis or osteochondritis

deformans juvenilis of the hip.

LIGAMENT: A band of fibrous tissue that connects bones or cartilages, serving to support or strengthen joints.

MORBIDITY: Pain, disability, and malfunctioning of a person brought about by disease.

MUSCLE FIBRIL: One of the units composing a muscle column, a number of which are grouped to form a muscle fiber.

MUSCLE SPASM: Involuntary convulsive muscular contraction.

MUSCULOSKELETAL: Describing the skeleton and the muscles.

MYALGIA: Muscular pain.

MYOSITIS: Nonsuppurative inflammation of muscle tissue.

OSTEOARTHROSIS: Osteoarthritis.

PLASMA PROTEIN: All proteins present in the blood plasma, including the immunoglobulins.

PLEURISY: Inflammation of the pleura, or the serous membrane covering the lungs.

POLYARTERITIS NODOSA: Connective tissue disease involving the small and medium sized arteries of the body. Symptoms include fever, weakness, weight loss, and arthritis.

POLYARTHRITIS: Inflammation of several joints.

POLYMYALGIA RHEUMATICA: A syndrome occurring most commonly in elderly persons, including pain and stiffness, particularly in the neck, back, pelvis, and shoulders.

POLYMYOSITIS: Inflammation of several muscles at once.

PROGRESSIVE SYSTEMIC SCLEROSIS: A generalized disorder of connective tissue characterized by inflammation, fibrosis and degenerative changes, and involving the skin, synovium, and certain internal organs.

PROSTHESIS: An artificial substitute for a missing body

GLOSSARY

part.

PROTEOGLYCAN: Complex carbohydrate-protein substance.

PSEUDOGOUT: Apparently hereditary and familial condition resembling gout, but with crystals of a calcium salt rather than urate crystals in the synovial fluid, leading to calcification and degenerative changes in cartilage; chondrocalcinosis.

PSORIASIS: Chronic, recurrent skin disease, frequently associated with chronic arthritis.

REITER'S SYNDROME: Combination of arthritis, conjunctivitis, and urethritis of unknown etiology.

RHEUMATIC DISEASES: Any of a number of diseases marked by inflammation of the connective tissue structures of the body, especially the muscles and joints.

RHEUMATIC FEVER: A nonsuppurative, acute, connective tissue disease which is a complication of Group A, streptococcal infections, and characterized by arthritis, sore throat and/or carditis, with residual heart disease a possible sequel.

RHEUMATISM: Any of a variety of disorders marked by inflammation, degeneration, or metabolic derangement of the connective tissue structures of the body.

RHEUMATOID ARTHRITIS: A chronic syndrome characterized by nonspecific inflammation of the peripheral joints, usually symmetrical with reference to the affected joint as well as to the right and left sides of the body, and resulting in progressive destruction of articular and periarticular structures.

RHEUMATOID FACTOR: A protein of high-molecular weight appearing in the serum of most patients with rheumatoid arthritis and detectable by serological tests.

SACROILIAC: A term that refers to the joint between the sacrum, a triangular bone at the lower end of the spine, and the ilium, the upper portion of the hip bone.

SCLERODERMA: Chronic disease of unknown cause, usually diffuse though sometimes localized, and characterized by fibrosis, rigidity, and thickening of the skin and subcutaneous tissues and by frequent involvement of internal organs; dermatosclerosis.

SLIPPED CAPITAL FEMORAL EPIPHYSIS: Dislocation of the epiphysis of the head of the femur causing a deformity of the hip.

SOMATOMEDIN: A blood protein factor.

SPONDYLITIS: Inflammation of the vertebrae.

STEROID: A group name for compounds that include sex and adrenocortical hormones. Synthetic steroids, like cortisone, are sometimes used in the treatment of arthritis.

SYNOVIAL FLUID: Transparent viscid fluid, resembling the white of egg, secreted by the synovial membrane contained in joint cavities, bursae, and tendon sheaths.

SYNOVIAL MEMBRANE: Joint lining formed of connective tissue; synovium.

SYNOVITIS: Inflammation of the synovial membrane.

SYSTEMIC LUPUS ERYTHEMATOSUS (SLE): Chronic inflammatory disease of unknown origin with clinical manifestations such as fever, rash, polyarthralgia and arthritis, polyserositis, and other blood, renal, neurologic and cardiac abnormalities.

TENDON: A fibrous cord by which a muscle is attached to a bone.

TENDONITIS: Inflammation of a tendon or of tendon-muscle attachments.

TRAUMATIC ARTHRITIS: Arthritis due to direct trauma to a joint and surrounding tissues.

URATE CRYSTAL: A crystal formed of any uric acid salt.

URIC ACID: An acid found in urine which can form crystals. An excessive amount of uric acid is found in the blood in gout.

VERTEBRAE: The bones of the spinal column.

Suggested Further Reading

Adams, Ruth, *The Complete Home Guide to All the Vitamins*, Larchmont Books, New York, N.Y.

Adams, Ruth and Frank Murray, *Is Low Blood Sugar Making You a Nutritional Cripple?*, Larchmont Books, New York, N.Y.

Adams, Ruth and Frank Murray, *Minerals: Kill or Cure?*, Larchmont Books, New York, N.Y.

Aikman, Lonnelle, *Nature's Healing Arts*, National Geographic Society, Washington, D.C.

Arehart-Treichel, Joan, *Trace Elements, How They Help and Harm Us,* Holiday House, New York, N.Y.

Aschner, Bernard, *Arthritis Can be Cured*, Arco Publications, New York City, N.Y.

Barnes, Broda O., and Lawrence Galton, *Hypothyroidism, the Unsuspected Illness*, Thomas Y. Crowell Co., New York, N.Y.

Bellew, Bernard A. and Joeva Galaz Bellew, *The Desert Yucca*, Spa City Graphics, Desert Hot Springs, Cal.

Berson, Dvera, with Sander Roy, *Pain-Free Arthritis*, Simon and Schuster, New York City, N.Y.

Blaine, Judge Tom, *Goodbye Allergies*, Citadel Press, 120 Enterprise Ave., Secaucus, N.J.

Campbell, Giraud W., *How to Control Arthritis*, Caravelle Books, New York, N.Y.

Childers, N. F. and G. M. Russo, *The Nightshades and*

Health, Somerset Publishers, Somerville, N.J. 08876.

Clark, Randolph Lee and Russell W. Cumley, *The Book of Health*, Jove Publications, Harcourt Brace Jovanovich, New York, N.Y.

Crain, Darrell C., *The Arthritis Handbook*, Arco Publishing Co., New York, N.Y.

Davis, Adelle, *Let's Get Well*, New American Library, New York, N.Y.

Dong, Colin H. and Jane Banks, *New Hope for the Arthritic*, Ballantine Books, New York, N.Y.

Ellis, John M. and James Presley, *Vitamin B₆, the Doctor's Report*, Harper and Row, New York, N.Y.

Fernie, W. T., *Meals Medicinal*, John Wright and Co., Bristol, England.

Fredericks, Carlton and Herbert Bailey, *Food Facts and Fallacies*, Arco Books, New York, N.Y.

Fredericks, Carlton, *High Fiber Way to Total Health*, Simon and Schuster, New York, N.Y.

Fredericks, Carlton, *Psycho-Nutrition*, Grosset and Dunlap, New York, N.Y.

Harris, Ben Charles, *The Compleat Herbal*, Larchmont Books, New York, N.Y.

Holvey, David N., Editor, *The Merck Manual*, Merck, Sharp and Dohme Research Laboratories, Rahway, N.J.

Hunter, Kathleen, *Health Foods and Herbs*, Arco Publications, New York, N.Y.

Hylton, William H., Editor, *The Rodale Herb Book*, Rodale Press, Emmaus, Pa.

Jayson, Malcolm I.V. and Allan St. J. Dixon, *Understanding Arthritis and Rheumatism*, Dell Publishing Co., New York, N.Y.

Kadans, Joseph, *Encyclopedia of Medicinal Herbs*, Arco Publishing Co., New York, N.Y.

Kaufman, William, *The Common Form of Joint Dysfunction: Its Incidence and Treatment*, E. L. Hildreth

SUGGESTED FURTHER READING

and Co., Brattleboro, Vt.

Kordel, Lelord, *Natural Folk Remedies*, G. P. Putnam's Sons, New York, N.Y.

Lucas, Richard, *Common and Uncommon Uses of Herbs for Healthful Living*, Arco Publishing Co., New York, N.Y.

Lucas, Richard, *Nature's Medicines*, Parker Publishing Co., West Nyack, N.Y.

Mességué, Maurice, *Way to Natural Health and Beauty*, Macmillan Publishing Co., New York, N.Y.

Millspaugh, Charles F., *American Medicinal Plants*, Dover Publications, New York, N.Y.

National Academy of Sciences, *Toxicants Occurring Naturally in Foods*, National Academy of Sciences, Washington, D.C.

Pauling, Linus, *Vitamin C and the Common Cold*, W. H. Freeman and Co., San Francisco, Cal.

Pfeiffer, Carl, *Mental and Elemental Nutrients*, Keats Publishing, Inc., New Canaan, Ct.

Hills, Hilda Cherry, *Good Food, Gluten-Free*, Keats Publishing, Inc., New Canaan, Ct.

Prasad, Ananda S., *Trace Elements in Human Health and Disease*, Volume I, Academic Press, New York, N.Y.

Roberts, Sam E., *Exhaustion, Causes and Treatment*, Rodale Press, Emmaus, Pa.

Roe, Daphne A., *Drug-Induced Nutritional Deficiencies*, The Avi Publishing Co., Westport, Ct.

Stone, Irwin, *The Healing Factor, Vitamin C Against Disease*, Grosset and Dunlap, New York, N.Y.

Underwood, E. J., *Trace Elements in Human and Animal Nutrition*, Academic Press, New York, N.Y.

Weiner, Michael A., *Earth Medicine-Earth Foods*, The Macmillan Co., New York, N.Y.

Williams, Roger J., *Nutrition Against Disease*, Bantam Books, New York, N.Y.

Williams, Roger J., *Nutrition in a Nutshell*, Doubleday and Co., Garden City, N.Y.

Williams, Roger J., *Physician's Handbook of Nutritional Science*, Charles C. Thomas, Springfield, Ill.

Wood, Curtis, Jr., *Overfed but Undernourished*, Tower Publications, New York, N.Y.

Yudkin, John, *Lose Weight, Feel Great*, Larchmont Books, New York, N.Y.

Yudkin, John, *Sweet and Dangerous*, Bantam Books, New York, N.Y.

Index

INDEX

INDEX

INDEX

INDEX

INDEX

INDEX

INDEX

INDEX

INDEX

INDEX

INDEX